TITLE PAGE

FOODS THAT FIGHT CANCER

A SECRET GUIDE THAT EXPOSE THE TRUTH ABOUT CANCER

JANE LORDSON

Copyrighted Material

This book or parts thereof may not be reproduced in any form whatsoever, store or transmitted by any means-electronic, photocopy, mechanical recording or otherwise without prior permission of the publisher.

Dedication

To all those who are currently having running battle with Cancer. Though the battle may look tough and insurmountable, but be aware that cancer is not a death sentence. You shall survive it!

Table of Content

''sometime in the future, nutrition will be the drugs for treating many diseases''

Introduction

Cancer is a dreaded disease worldwide. While modern medicine is still struggling to proffer solution to the disease, mounting evidence shows that we may not need to wait extensively for medical solution, as study has discovered that the foods we eat weigh heavily in the war against cancer.

As researchers continue in their war against the disease, many nutritionists have begun to shift attention to what could be the most potent weapon against cancer to date: diet.

Diet has been discovered to be the least expensive and easiest way of reducing the risk of cancer. Many common foods contain antioxidant substances which inhibit the growth of cancer in human. Most expert agree that cancer fighting diet should be dominant in plant- based diet and diet high in saturated fat should be avoided.

Study has concluded by notable nutritionists that various plant based food substances listed in this book are healthy, high in antioxidants with excellent cancer fighting agents.

It is interesting to note that most of these plant based diet can be consume in their natural form, while some others may be eaten as snacks, cookies, salad, spices to food, cook or boil.

Cancer: An insight

Cancer is a general term for a group of diseases that can develop in almost any area of the body part. One major feature of the disease is the rapid growth of abnormal cells which later outgrow beyond their usual boundaries, and later invade adjoining body parts and spread to other organs in the body structure. The latter process is refers to as metastasizing. The major cause of death from cancer is Metastases.

It is important to know that what we eat can actually affect a greater part of our health, including risk of developing chronic ailment like diabetes, cancer and heart related disease.

Cancer development has been established to be greatly influenced by various foods we consumed.

It is pertinent to note that higher intake of some foods could be associated with high risk of exposure to certain diseases (including cancer) because of their composition of various degrees of unhealthy compound elements that are harmful to human's health. On the other hand, some foods actually contained healthy compounds that are beneficial in reducing the growth of those diseases.

Cancer has been identified as the second most common causes of death globally after heart disease. It is responsible for over 9 million deaths globally in 2018 alone, and 1 out of 6 deaths are as a result of cancer. While cancer is a deadly disease, it is good to know that a significant percentage of new diagnosed can be cured when detected early. Though, some cancer can develop completely without any major signs. Taking note and being conscious of cancer symptoms can be a life saver as early detection can be a key in the management and treatment of the disease.

What Are Signs and Symptoms of Cancer?

Cancer sometime exhibits no traces, signs or symptoms, but most of the complaint can be explained by harmless condition to a large extent. However, it is advisable to see a doctor for further evaluation if there is a persistent of certain symptoms over a long period of time.

Symptoms and signs of cancer are different depending on the part of the body affected. Some common signs and symptoms associated with, though not limited to cancer alone include:

> Breast discharge or lump:

> Special attention should be paid to breast lump as they need to be investigated from time to time. Though not all breast lumps are cancerous. In some cases, discharge from breast may be considered normal but some forms of discharge may be a symptom of cancer which may require further examination. It is highly recommended for women to consider conducting monthly breast examinations.

➤ Persistent Cough/ blood-tinged saliva:

Persistent cough lasting more than a month with blood in the mucus could be symptoms of cancer of the long, neck and head.

➤ Discharge or unusual vaginal bleeding:

Bloody discharge or unusual vagina bleeding may be a warning symptom of cancer of the uterus. It is highly recommended for women to be examined when they notice bleeding between periods or after intercourse. Routine bleeding that lasts for days or that is heavier than usual need medical examination. A pap smear should be included in every woman's medical routine.

➤ A change in bowel habits:

Changes in bowel habits are mostly associated to fluid intake and diet. Sometimes, cancer tends to exhibits a continuous sign of diarrhea. Some people living with have feeling of bowel movement and they still have the same feeling even after they have had that bowel movement. Medical evaluation is greatly required if this types of abnormal bowel complaints persist for days.

> Traces of Blood in the stool:

Medical attention should be sought for traces of blood in the stool. Hemorrhoids are common and often caused rectal bleeding, but sometimes it may exist with cancer. Thus, it is advisable to see a doctor even when you have hemorrhoids that you consider harmless.

More cancer warning signs

> Weight loss

> Blood loss

> Fever

> Skin changes

> Night sweats

- Pain and tiredness

- Digestive changes

- Persistent, unexplained muscle or joint pain

- Lumps in the testicles

- Change in the urination

- Unexplained anemia

- Non-healing sores

- Hoarseness

- Difficulty swallowing

- Unexplained bleeding and or nursing

Most common cancers

Based on the study conducted by NCI, the most common types of cancer in the United States are the following;

- Breast cancer

- Kidney cancer

➢ Bladder cancer

➢ Liver cancer

➢ Melanoma

➢ Colon and rectal cancer

➢ Leukemia

➢ Thyroid cancer

➢ Lung cancer

➢ Prostate cancer

➢ Pancreatic cancer

➢ Non-melanoma cancer

Among all of these, lung and breast cancer has been identified as the most common, with more than 200,000 Americans diagnosed each year. In comparison to thyroid, liver and pancreatic that has fewer than 60,000 yearly reported cases.

Cancer myths and misconceptions

Some cancer myths and misconceptions are nothing but just a fairytales that created needless worry and hinder prevention and treatment decisions. Some of these myths are highlighted below:

➤ Cancer is a death sentence:

There is a common believe that once you have been diagnosed of cancer, you have gotten your death sentence. The important point to note here is that how long a cancer patient will live depend on many factors like; availability of effective treatment method, whether the cancer is slow or fast growing, to what extent has the cancer spread in the body and so on. The good news is that the rate of death from cancer has drastically reduced due to improved medical care.

➤ Sugar consumption will worsen the cancer condition:

Though it has been established that cancer cells consume more glucose than normal cells but no studies has proven that stopping sugar consumption will shrink cancer or make cancer disappear.

➤ Cancer is contagious:

Cancer is generally not a contagious disease that can easily be spread from one person to another. The only exception to this case is the issue of organ or tissue transplant. A receiver of tissue or organ from a donor with history of cancer in the past may be at risk of developing a transplant related cancer in the future.

➤ Cell phone cause cancer:

Cell phone emits low frequency energy harmless to gene, while cancer is caused by genetic mutations. Thus, the assertion that phones cell cause cancer is not true.

➤ Anti-perspirants and deodorants cause cancer:

No study has found chemical composition present in antiperspirants and deodorants with changes in breast tissue. Thus, to a large extent, it does not cause cancer.

Top 5 Cancer Causing Foods

1. Microwave Popcorn:

    This food is a major debate in relation to lung cancer around the world. From the chemically-lined bag, the contents and to the kernels and oil that is probably of a GMOs origin and the toxic fumes called diacetyl, which is released from the artificial butter flavoring makes microwaves popcorn toxic and a risk for human health. However, organic popcorn is safer and healthier for consumption.

2. Canned Foods:

    Most canned foods are lined with bisphenol-A, a chemical that has been clinically proven to alter rat brain cells.BPA is also present in most water lines, many plastic goods, dental composites and thermal paper. Therefore, it is advisable to stick to frozen or fresh vegetables with no additives than most canned foods.

3. Grilled Red Meat:

    Grilled red meat has a tendency of releasing harmful chemical called heterocyclic aromatic amines which occur when red meat is grilled to the point of well-done. It is safer boiling, baking or using skillet method for your meat than grilling them.

4. Refined Sugar:

Mutated cancer cells thrive well on sugar, little wonder that oncologists are now using diabetes medication to fights cancer cells. High fructose corn syrup (HFCS) and some other refined sugars are part of a major cancer causing food. They are major insulin spikes that aid the rapid growth and development of cancer cells.

5. Hydrogenated Oils:

These vegetable oils are chemically based in nature and are packed with unhealthy omega-6 fats which have been established to alter cell membranes structure. Americans are one of the top consumers of hydrogenated oil, thus, this explain the high rate of cancer in that part of the world.

Tips to Help Prevent Cancer

➢ Eliminate tobacco usage:

Tobacco usage increases your cancer risk. Tobacco has been identified as a suspect for various forms of cancer-including mouth cancer, lung cancer, throat cancer, bladder cancer, larynx pancreas and kidney cancer. Exposure to smoke can also increase the risk of cancer, especially lung cancer.

> ➤ Eat healthy and stay healthy:

Consider incorporating more of natural fruits and vegetables into your diets. Eat lighter, avoid obesity and limit your alcohol consumption.

> ➤ Consume wholly organic foods if possible.

> ➤ Always go for fresh organic product, raw or frozen if available in your area.

> ➤ Consider going for non-starchy vegetables and if you must eat animal products, ensure they are grass-fed. Also, stick to quality oils like olive oil, ghee and coconut oil.

> ➤ Reduce or eliminate grains and sugar consumption. Sugar of plant or insect origin is safer.

Sticking to these simple tips will not only helps in lowering your cancer risk, it will also aid you in maintain healthy living and promote general well-being.

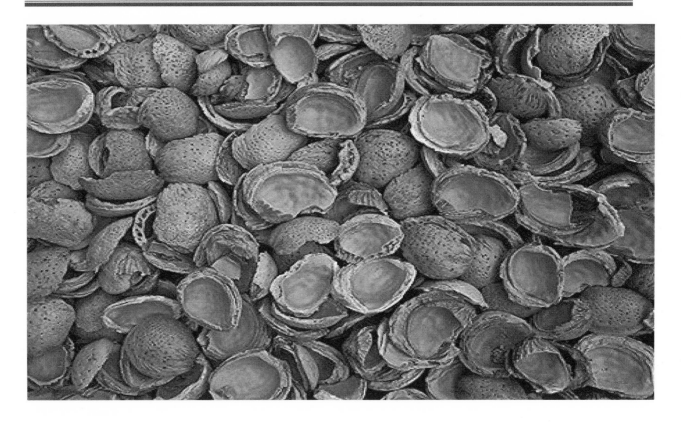

Almonds

Almonds are a very rich in vitamin E, biotin, manganese, and copper. *Almonds* are also source of riboflavin (vitamin B2), magnesium, and phosphorus. Interestingly, one-quarter cup of *almonds* have about 11 grams of fat, while about seven grams is heart-friendly and monounsaturated fat

Juice can be extracted from Almonds by soaking. To soak them, simply fill it up with ordinary water in a glass or bowl container overnight or for at least 12 hours. Then drain and refrigerate. The Almonds juice extract is particularly good in combating cancer and some other ailment. A glass cup a day is enough to get the best result.

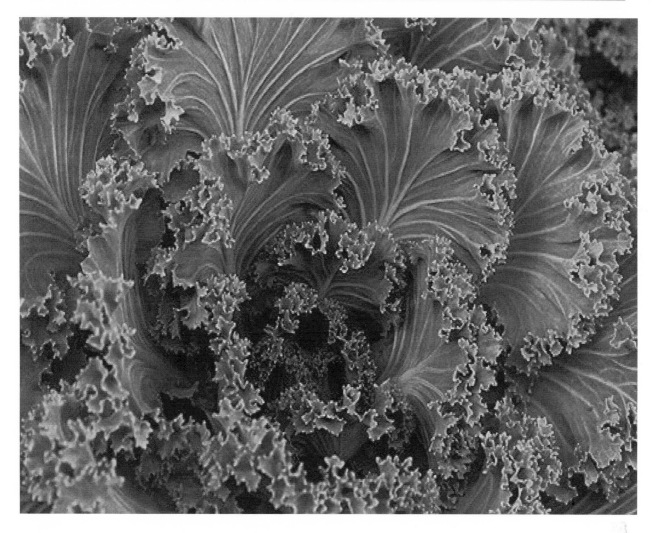

Kale

Kale is incredibly low *calorie* veggie and ranked among the most nutrient packed foods in the universe.

Kale contains many powerful antioxidants that are beneficial to health.

Extensive study shows that kale is a perfect source of vitamin K, vitamin A, vitamin C, copper and manganese. Also, it is an excellent source of fiber, vitamin B2, vitamin E, vitamin B6, calcium and potassium; and a rich source of magnesium, iron, vitamin B1, vitamin B3, omega-3 fats, protein, phosphorus and *foliates*.

To get the best out of kale, make it into a salad, chips, put it in the soup, or in a burger.

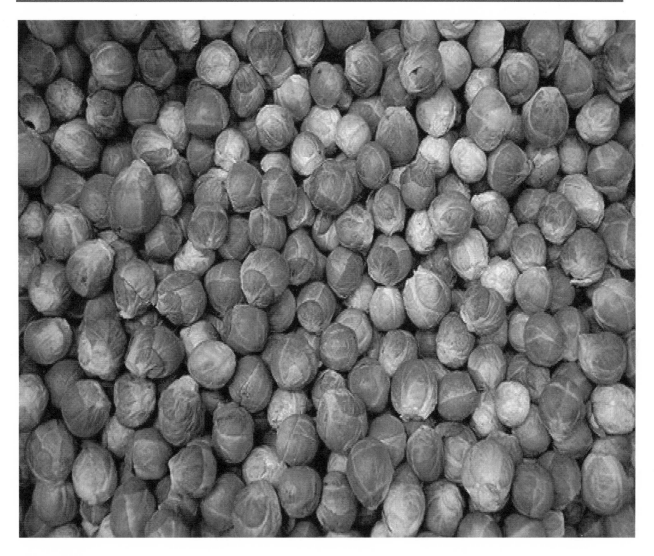

Sprouts

Sprouts are a strong antioxidant veggie which can help us fight chronic diseases through a variety of *nutrient benefits*. It is also an excellent source of Phosphorus and Potassium , Protein, pantothenic Acid, Nacin, Thiamin, Vitamin B6, Iron, Magnesium, , and a very good source of Riboflavin, *Dietary* Fiber, Copper and Manganese , Vitamin C and Vitamin K,

Sprouts can be added to sandwiches in place of lettuce, and can also be made into salad.

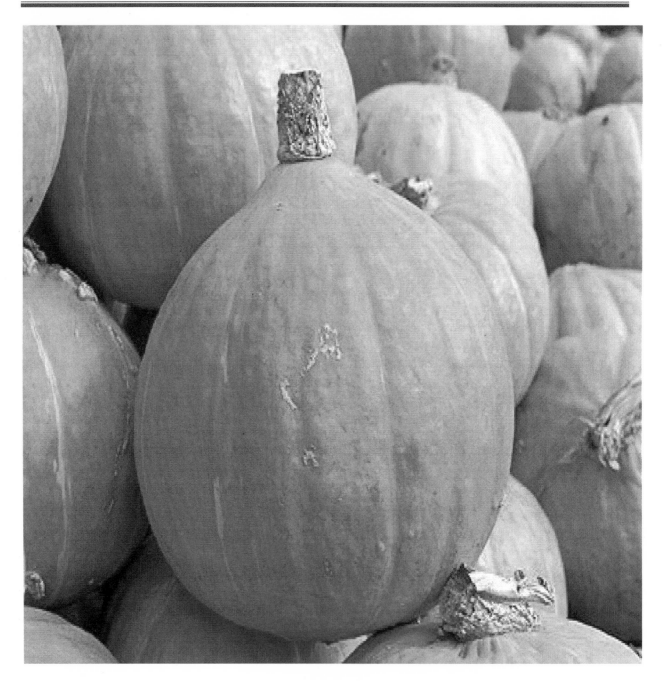

Pumpkins

Pumpkin is one of the popular vegetables densely rich in antioxidants and vitamins such as vitamins-A and vitamins C. It is an excellent source of protein, minerals and omega-3 fatty acids. To get the best out of pumpkin, it can be process into *Pumpkin* Snacks, bake into bread, snacks, Blend into a *pumpkin* smoothie, also as candied *pumpkin*. A few bites of pumpkins is strong enough to wade off diseases.

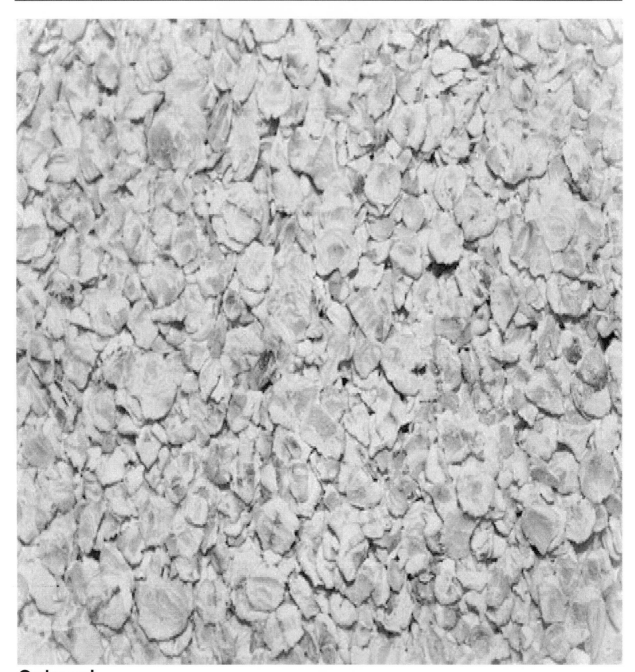

Oatmeal

Oats is a excellent food with a well-balanced *nutritional* composition. One serving thirty grams of oats contains about 117 *calories*. In weight, raw oats are 66% carbohydrates, 11% fiber, 7% fat and 17% protein.

This food is easy fantastically easy to prepared. To get the best out of oats, it can be dried and turned into powder to be added to tea or coffee.

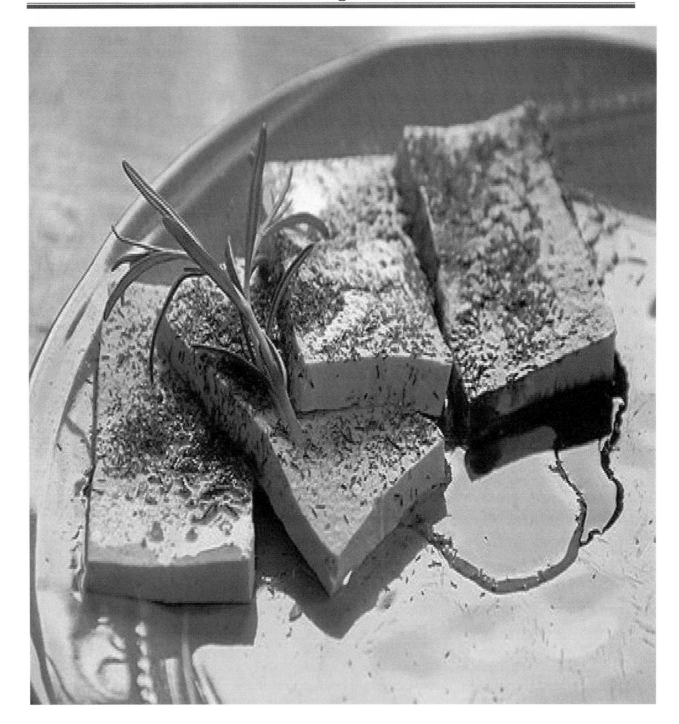

Tofu

Tofu is a great source of calcium, manganese, copper, selenium, protein and phosphorus. In addition, *tofu* is a good source of magnesium, omega-3 fatty acids, zinc iron and vitamin B1.Tofu is useful in treating many ailments and diseases.

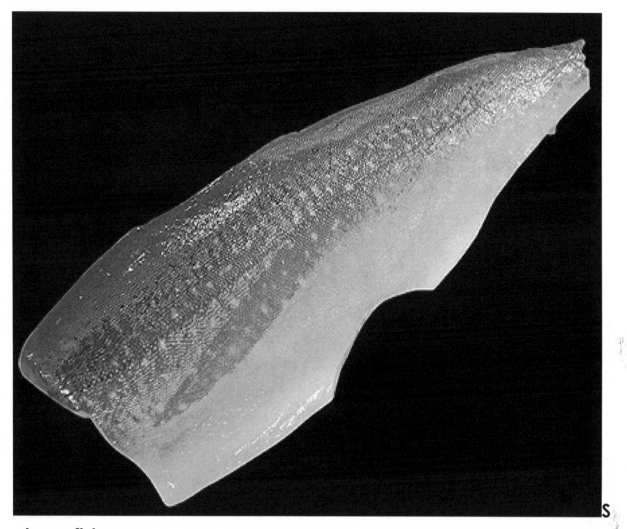

almon fish

Salmon is densely rich in B vitamins. Study has shown that a cooked portion of wild Atlantic salmon gives (48%) 0.828 milligrams of the recommended daily value, for vitamin B-2 and 17.13 milligrams of vitamin B-3 (84%) of the DV. These vitamins are vital for energy metabolism and nervous system function. Vitamin B-6 helps break down stored energy. Furthermore, vitamin B-6 is important for protein metabolism and regulates body functions. Vitamin B-12 is vital for energy metabolism, aiding proper function of the nervous system and forming new cells to combat diseases.

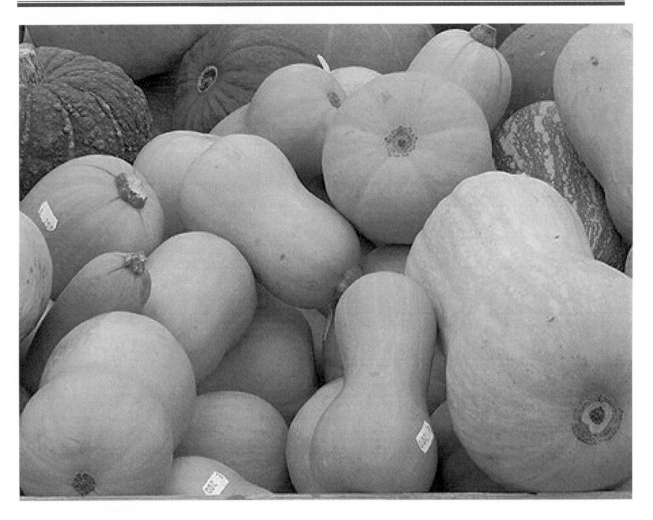

Winter squash

Winter squash is a major source of immune-supportive vitamin A in its natural form. It is also an excellent source of vitamin C, vitamins B6, *dietary* fiber, manganese and copper and also a good source of potassium, foliate, vitamin B2, vitamin K.

Squash is easy to cook. To cook winter squash, Place the squash halves, cut-side up, on a baking sheet. Cover the flesh with oil or butter and season with pepper, salt, and little sugar, maple syrup, or orange juice. Flip the squash over and roast them for 40 to 45 minutes in a preheated 400 degrees F (200 degrees C) oven. This can be eating as a snack.

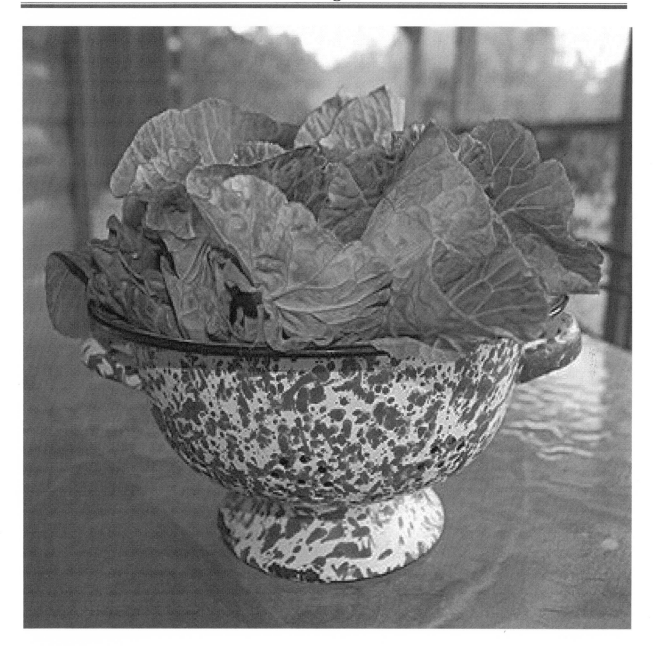

Collard green

Collard greens are very good source of vitamin K, vitamin A (in the form of carotenoids), manganese, vitamin C, *dietary* fiber and calcium. Also, *collard greens* are rich source of vitamin B1, vitamin B6 and iron,

Collard juice is a good way of getting most nutrient out of Collard. The juice can be extracted by boiling. One full cup of boiled *collard greens* have 63 *calories*, 5 grams of protein, 1 gram of fat, and 11 grams of carbohydrate, 8 grams of fiber and 1 gram of sugar.

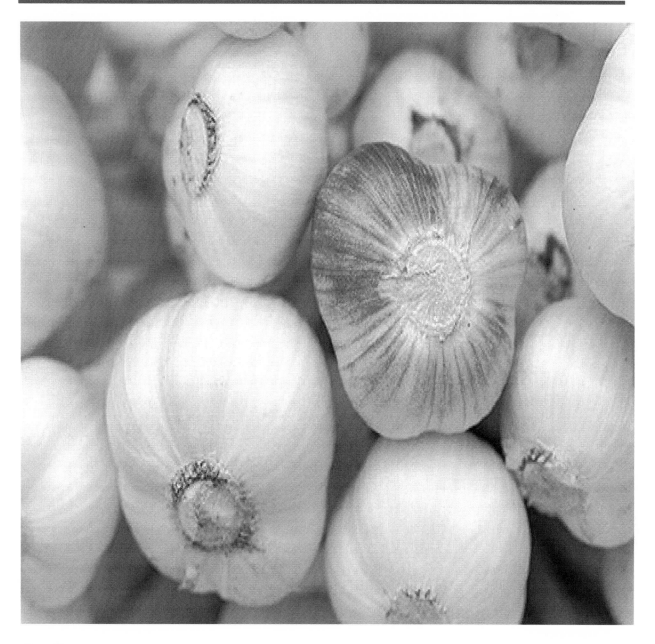

Garlic

Garlic is a very rich source of minerals and vitamins that are essential for good health. A bulb of garlic is densely packed with potassium, iron, calcium, magnesium, manganese, zinc, and selenium. Selenium is a heart-friendly mineral and is an essential for antioxidant enzymes in the body. Garlic juice and powder are excellently good in treating blood pressure, cancer and many ailments.

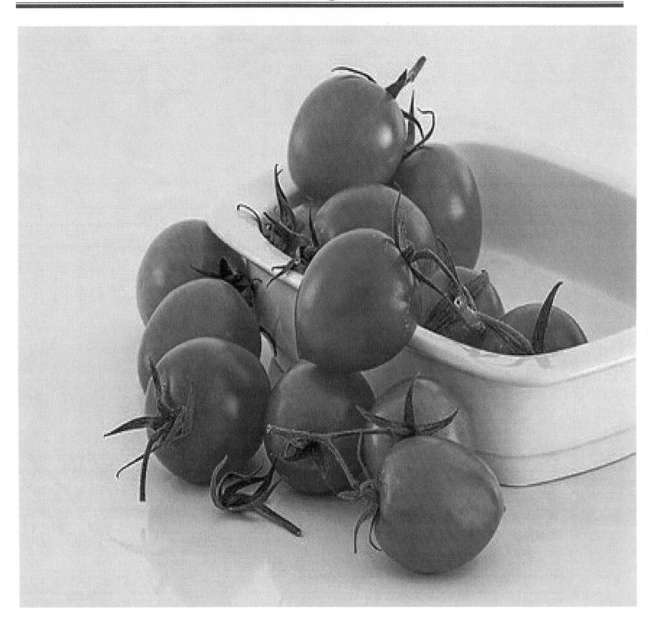

Tomatoes

Tomatoes consumption is good way of reducing heart diseases, cancer and many more ailments. It is a major *dietary* source of the lycopene which is an antioxidant. Lycopene, has been linked to many health *benefits*. They are also a great source of vitamin C, potassium, folate and vitamin K. It can be consumed fresh as salad or added to soup.

Carbohydrates: 3.9 g   **Protein**: 0.9 g
Calories: 18   **Fiber**: 1.2 g

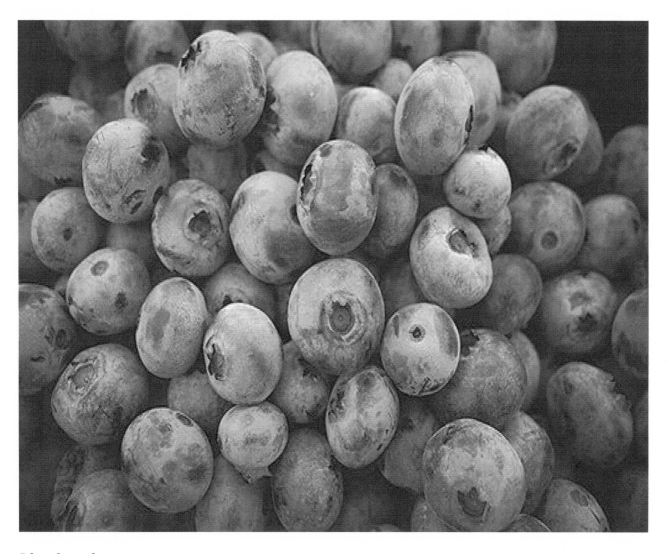

Blueberries

Blueberries are rich in vitamins C, K and manganese with strong antioxidants. *Blueberries* are also rich in fiber and copper with a very low Saturated Fat, Cholesterol and Sodium. It is also a good source of *Dietary* Fiber. *Blueberries* are an antioxidant-packed fruit that have many health benefits and ability to combat many ailments.

Carbs: 14.5 g   **Sugar**: 10 g

Protein: 0.7 g   **Calories**: 57

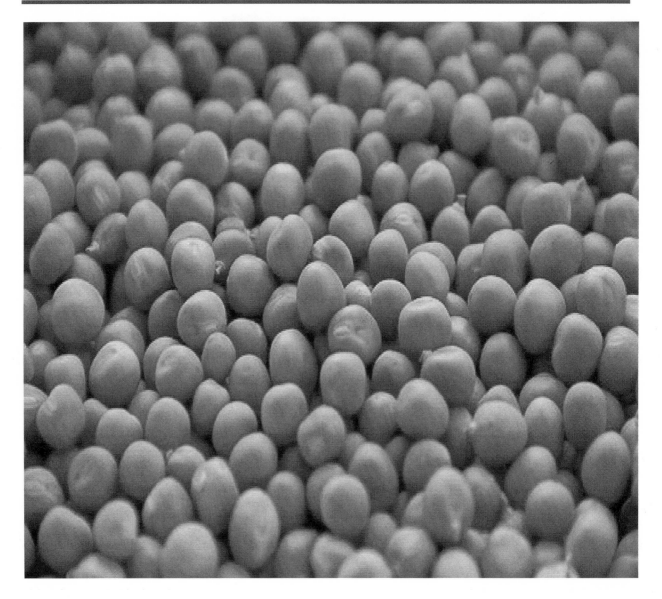

Peas

Peas are low in Saturated Fat, sodium and Cholesterol. It is a major source of *Protein*, Niacin, Vitamin A, Riboflavin, Vitamin B6, dietary fiber, Magnesium, Phosphorus and Copper, and a great source of Vitamin C, Vitamin K, Manganese and Thiamin. Peas' consumption can be used to control blood pressure, treat cancer and many more diseases. It can be cook or used as a salad.

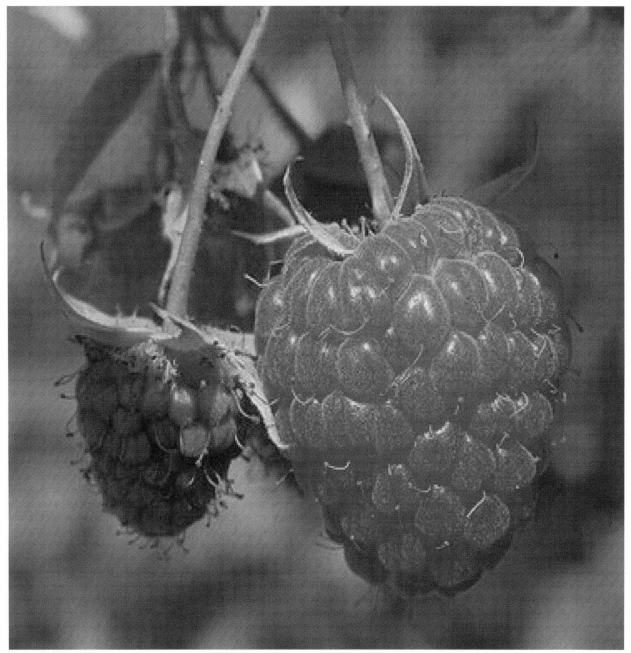

Raspberry

Raspberries are a major source of vitamins K, copper, biotin, vitamin E, magnesium, omega-3 fatty acids, potassium and dietary fiber. It is also good source of vitamin C and manganese.

Raspberry is very rich in antioxidants, with highest ORAC *values* and considered as one of the wonder and super fruits.

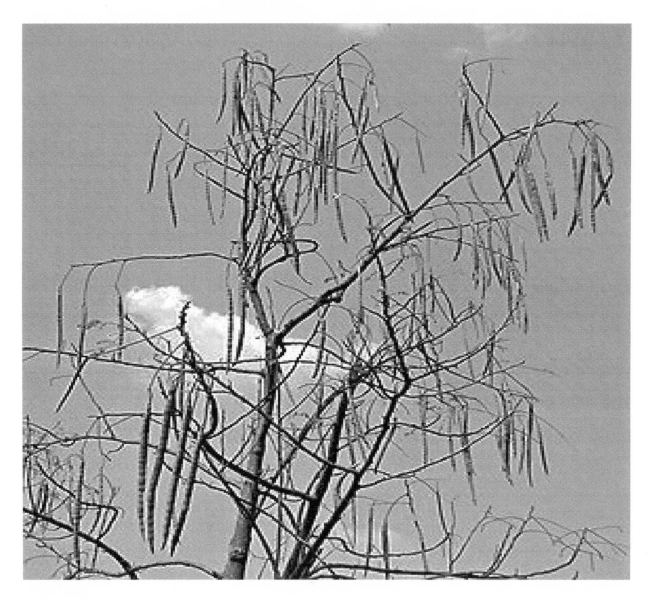

Moringa

The *Moringa* is also known as oleifera. It is a great source of *nutrition*, especially in areas where other food sources are deficient. Moringa Leaves and seeds are full of essential disease-preventing nutrients. The oleifera' seeds and leaves have been successfully used in treating blood sugar, blood pressure, cancer and many more. The seeds and leaves can be process into powder or soak in a clean water to extract the juice. A glass cup of oleifera juice a day is enough to get optimum benefits.

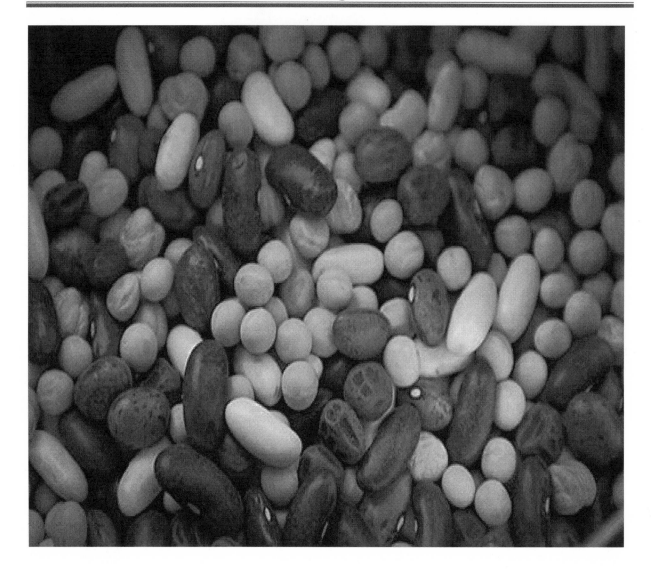

Soya beans

Soya beans are a Cholesterol and Sodium low food. It has a good source of *Dietary* Fiber, Vitamin K, Iron, Magnesium, Phosphorus and Copper. Soya beans are a very good source of manganese, phosphorus, protein, iron, omega-3 fatty acids, *dietary* fiber, vitamin B2, magnesium, vitamin K and potassium. The soya beans can be cook or roasted and eaten as snacks.

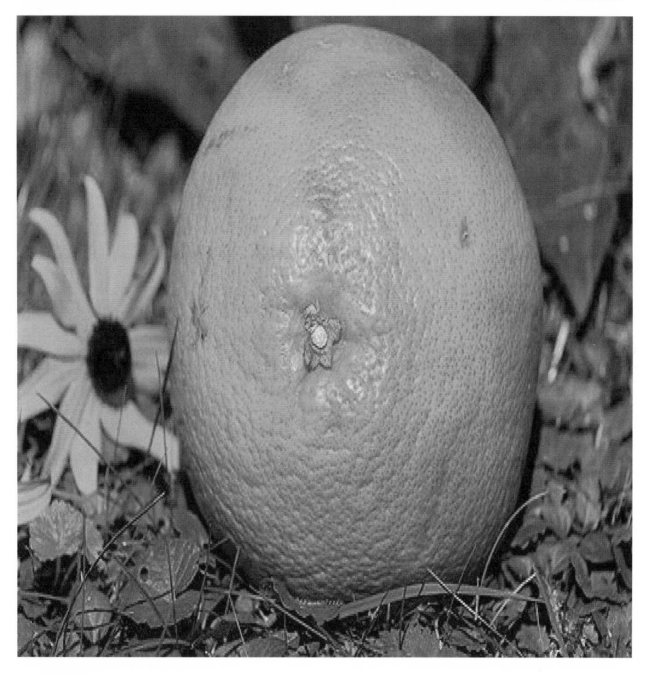

Grapefruit

Grapefruit is a great source of vitamin A (carotenoids) and *vitamin* C. It is also rich in pantothenic acid, copper, dietary fiber, *potassium*, biotin and vitamin B1. Grape contains phytochemicals including liminoids and *lycopene*. *Grapefruit* has low *calories*, consists of just 42 *calories* per 100 g. The skin of the fruit contains a very strong antioxidant that helps in fighting many diseases.

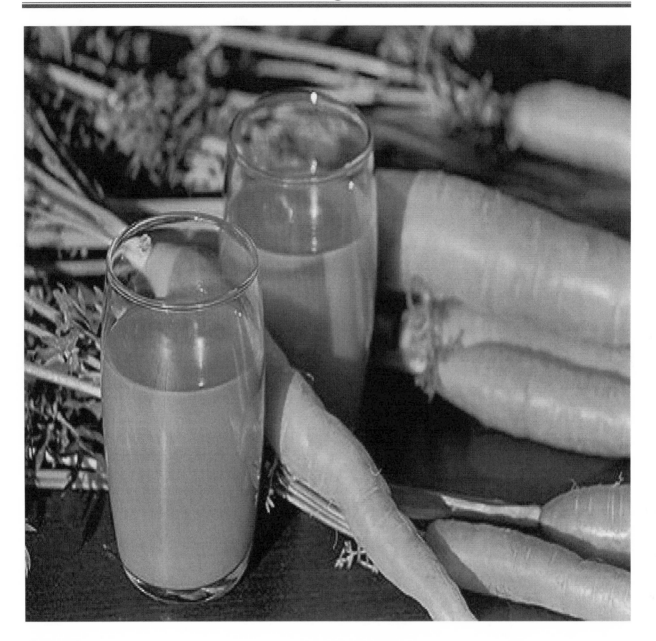

Carrot

The *carrot* also known as Daucus carota is a root vegetable that is perfect for health. It is reddish, tasty and naturally *nutritious*. *Carrots* are a rich source of beta-carotene, fiber, vitamin K, potassium and antioxidants (1). *Carrots* have a number of health benefits and serves as antioxidant.

Carbs: 9.6 g   **Calories**: 41

Protein: 0.9 g   **Fat**: 0.2 g

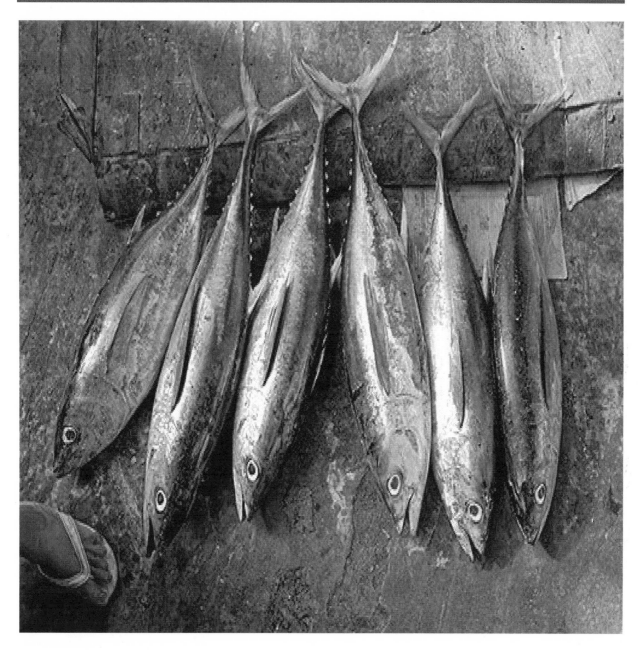

Tuna Fish

Tuna fish is a perfect source of selenium, vitamin B3 (niacin), vitamin B12, vitamin B6, and *protein*. It is a very good source of phosphorus as well as a good source of vitamin B1 (thiamin), vitamin B2 (riboflavin), vitamin D, and the minerals potassium, iodine, and magnesium. The oil in Tuna is a great balm in treating many diseases.

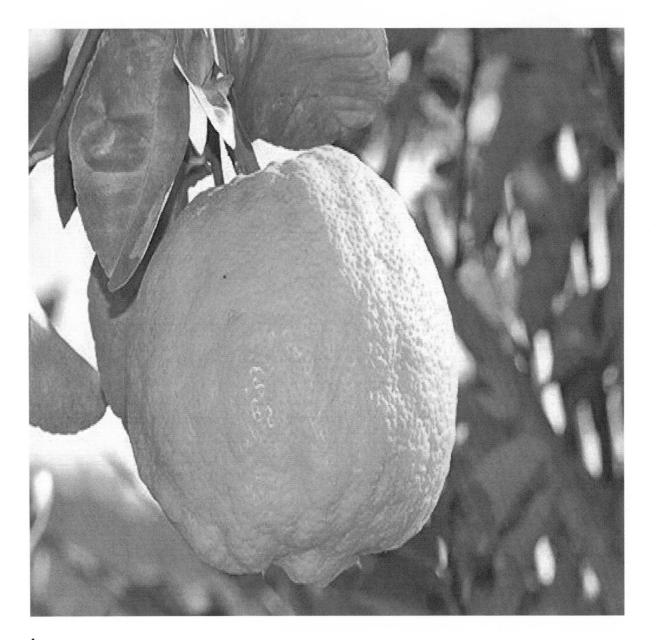

Lemon

Citric contain a natural preservative which aids in the digestion process, destroy harmful bacteria and helps to dissolve kidney stone. Lemons are good source of vitamin-C and it gives around 88% of daily recommended intake. Its strong antioxidant presence is greatly beneficial in fighting diseases such cancer, weight loss and many more.

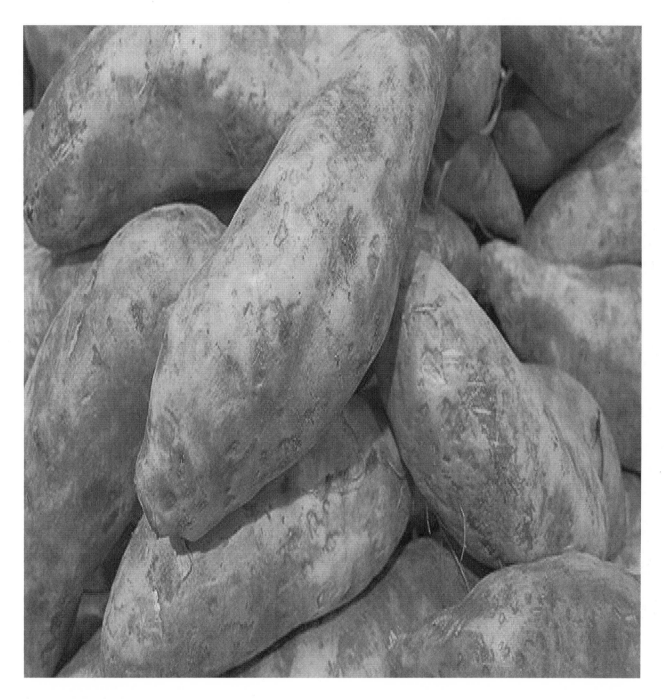

Sweet Potatoes

Sweet potatoes are densely rich in *vitamin A* (in the form of *beta-carotene*). They are also an excellent source of *vitamin C*, manganese, copper and *vitamin B6*. In addition, they are a perfect source of potassium, *dietary fiber*, niacin, *vitamin* B1, *vitamin* B2, phosphorus with a strong ability to wade off some chronic diseases.

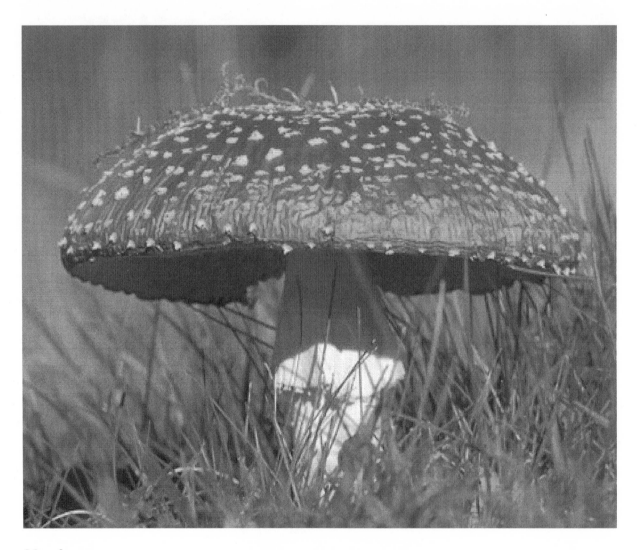

Mushroom

Mushrooms are flamboyant plant rich in minerals like copper, selenium and *phosphorus*. They are also a good source of B vitamins including vitamin B2, niacin, potassium, *zinc*, vitamin B1 and manganese. The antioxidant presence in mushroom makes it healthy and strong for many diseases and ailment. The plant can be cook or added to a bowl of soup.

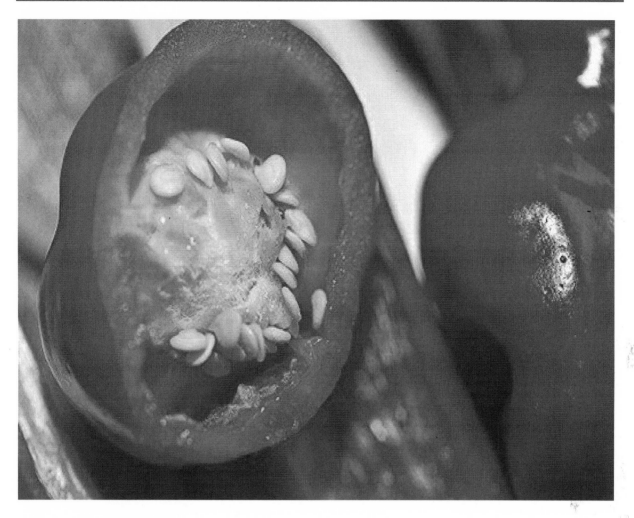

Cayenne Pepper

Cayenne pepper is a tasty spice very low in Cholesterol and Sodium. It is an excellent source of Riboflavin, Niacin, Iron, Magnesium and Potassium, and a perfect source of *Dietary* Fiber, Vitamin A, Vitamin C, Vitamin E, Vitamin K, Vitamin B6 and Manganese. It is useful in treating diseases like cancer and others.

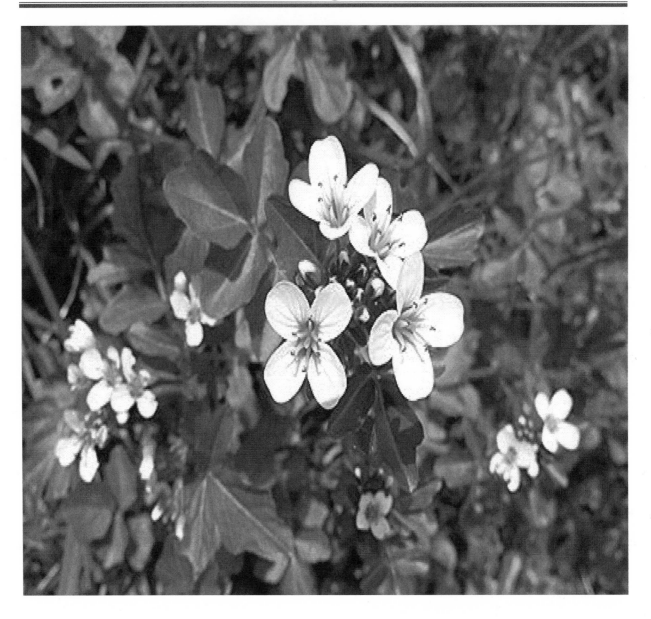

Watercress

Watercress is a cruciferous vegetable containing glucosinolates, phytochemicals that have anticancer effects. Good intake of these compounds has been shown to prevent breast, lung, colorectal, head and neck, and prostate cancers. The plant is also rich in lutein and other essential vitamins.

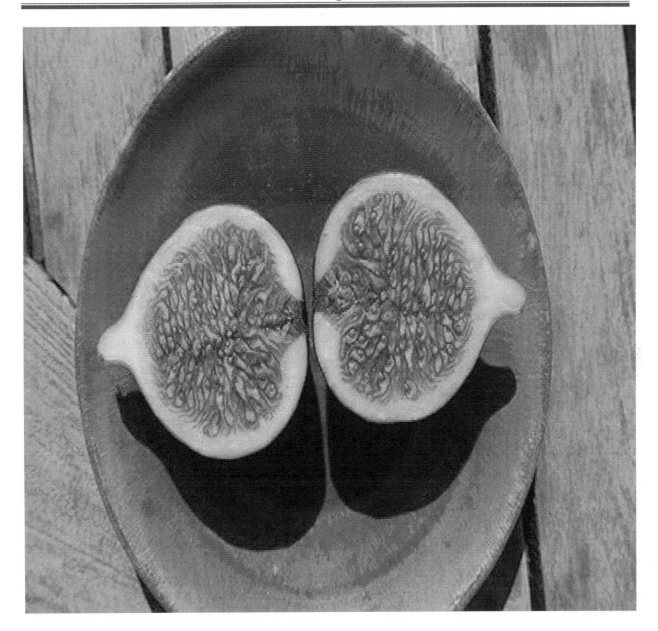

Figs

Figs are rich in fiber and a great source of essential minerals, like magnesium, manganese, calcium , copper, and potassium , as well as vitamins, principally K and B6.Figs can be used to treat cases like high blood pressure, cancer etc.

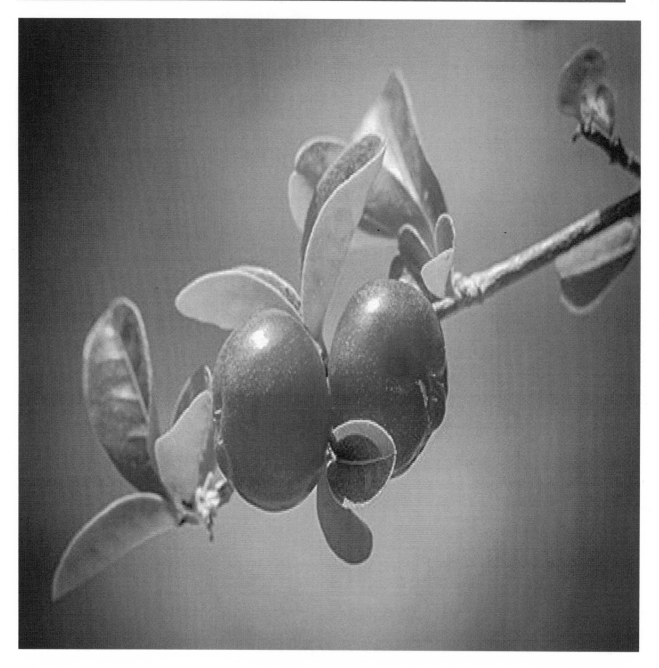

Cherry

Cherry fruits are bright red delicious fruits loaded with essential *nutrients.*

This fruit is very low in cholesterol, sodium and Saturated Fat. It is a great source of *Dietary* Fiber and Vitamin C. Sweet Cherries are effective in cancer prevention and treatment and in treating other diseases.

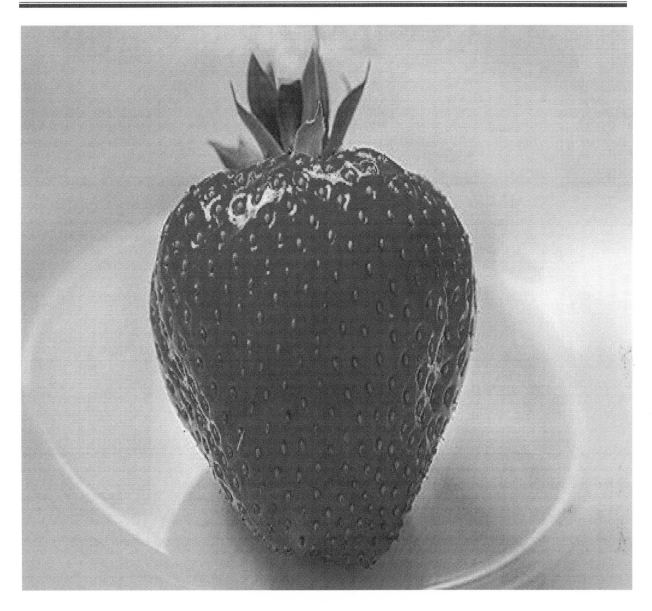

Strawberry

Strawberries are a juicy, bright red in color with a sweet flavor. They are rich in vitamin C and manganese, and also have foliate (B9) and potassium.

Strawberries are antioxidants rich plant, and have benefits for heart health and blood sugar control, cancer treatment and many more. It can be consumed raw and fresh and can also be used in a jams, jellies and desserts.

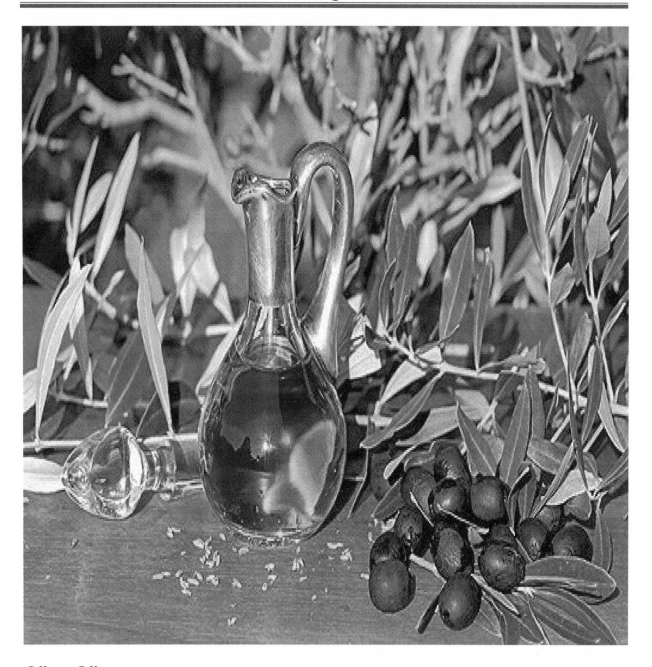

Olive Oil

Olive oil is excellent edible *oil* in terms of stability and degree of palatability. It is dense in energy; 100 g *oil* gives about 884 *calories*. It is in high mono-unsaturated fatty acids which make it as one of the best and healthiest *oil* safe human for consumption.

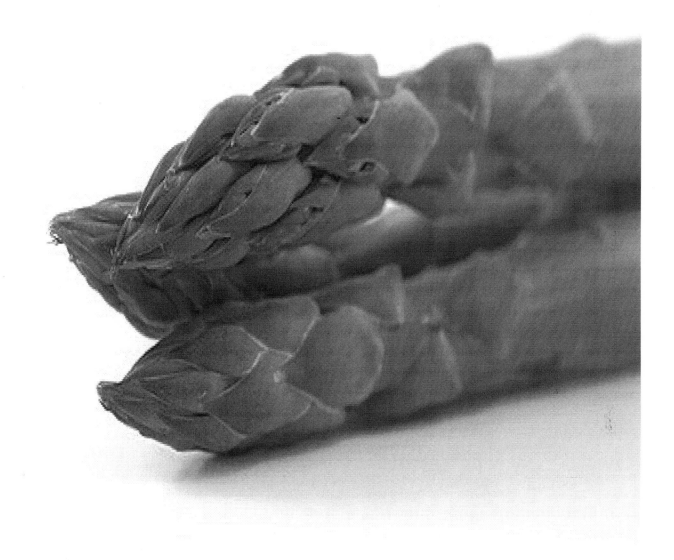

Asparagus

Asparagus is a rich source of vitamin K, copper, vitamin B2, vitamin C, and vitamin E. It is an excellent source of *dietary* fiber, manganese, phosphorus, niacin, potassium, vitamin A, zinc, iron, protein and vitamin B6.

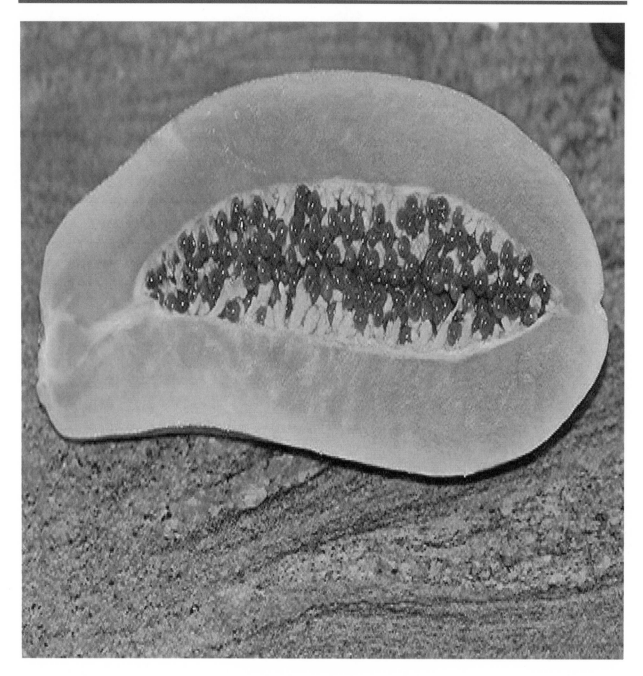

Papaya

Papaya is also known as pawpaw. It is very low in Saturated Fat, low in Cholesterol and Sodium. It is also a perfect source of *Dietary* Fiber and Potassium. Papaya rich sources of antioxidant *nutrients* includes; carotenes, vitamin C, flavonoids, foliate and pantothenic acid as well as the minerals, potassium, copper, and magnesium; and fiber.

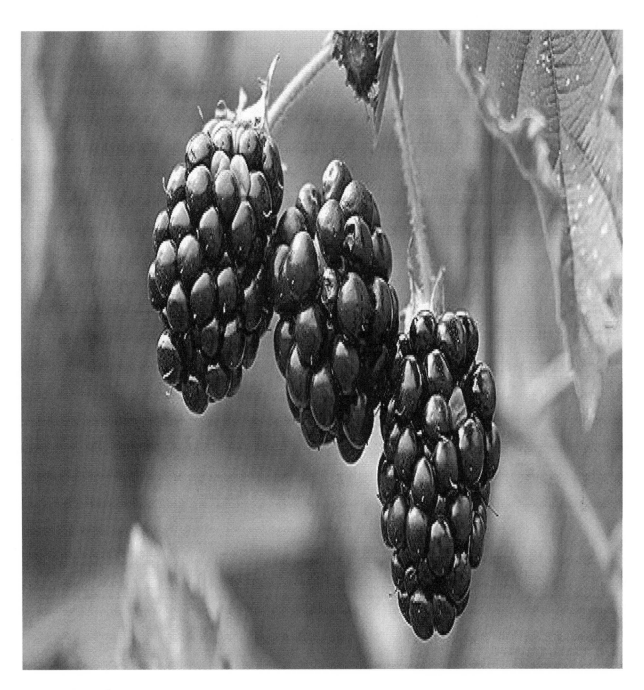

Blackberries

Blackberries are very low in Saturated Fat, Cholesterol and Sodium. It is also a perfect source of Vitamin E , Magnesium, Potassium and Copper, and an excellent source of Dietary Fiber, *Vitamin C*, Vitamin K and Manganese.

The nutrient compositions of blackberries are numerous. They are dense with *vitamin C.* and are excellent source of soluble and insoluble fiber.

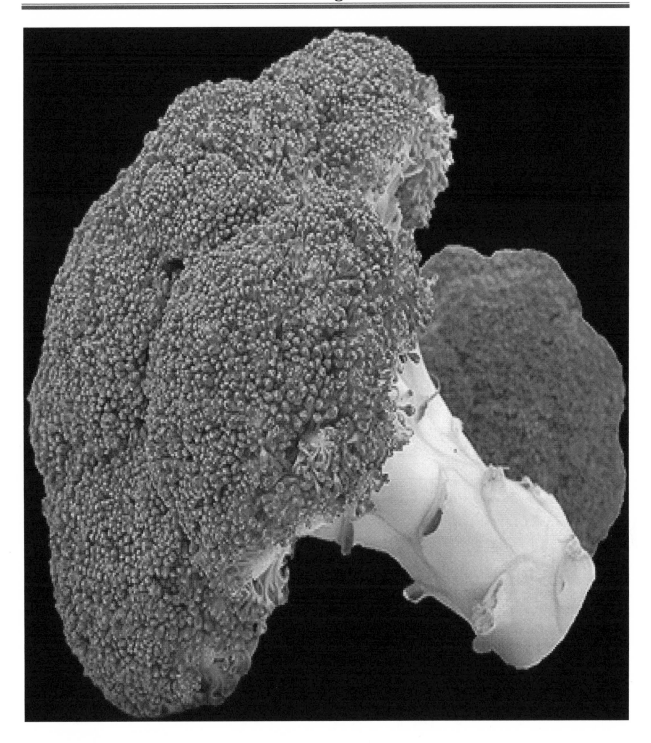

Broccoli

Broccoli is a natural source of Protein, Vitamin E , Thiamin, Riboflavin, Calcium, Iron, Magnesium, Phosphorus and Selenium. It is also a good source of *Dietary* Fiber, and Vitamin like; Vitamin A, Vitamin C, Vitamin K, Vitamin B6, Foliate, Potassium and Manganese.

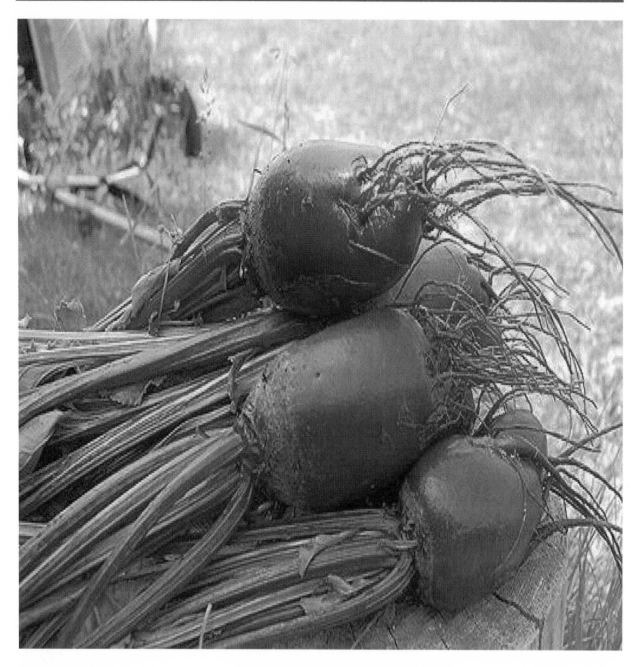

Turnips

Turnips are a very low Saturated Fat and Cholesterol food. It has a perfect source of Vitamin B6, Calcium, Phosphorus and Manganese, and a good source of *Dietary* Fiber, Vitamin C and Potassium. Its medicinal value is not in doubt.

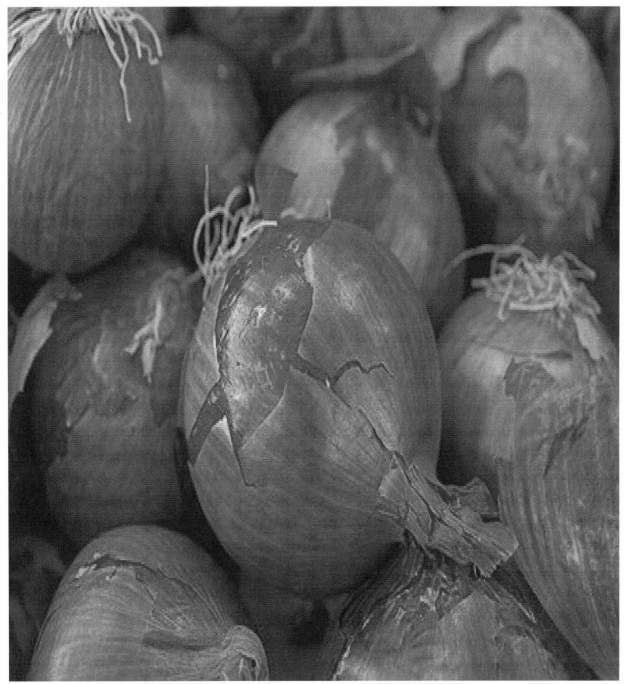

Onions

Onions is a bulb food with multi layers of health *benefits*. Active *nutrients* in *onions* helps nourishing the heart, reduce inflammation, and fight cancer. Onions are perfect source of biotin, manganese, vitamin B6, copper, vitamin C, *dietary fiber*, phosphorus, *potassium*, *foliate* and vitamin B1.

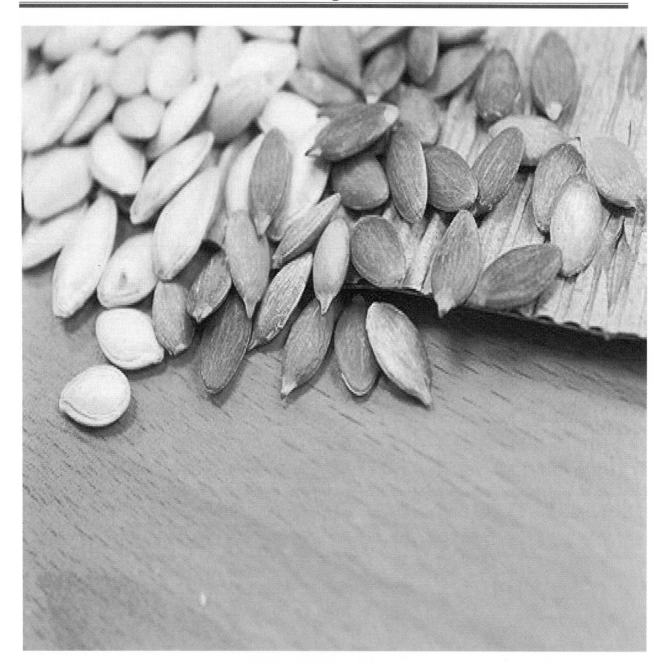

Pumpkin seeds

Pumpkin seeds contain a wide variety of *nutrients* ranging from magnesium and manganese to copper, protein and zinc, *pumpkin seeds* are *nutritional* giant houses in a very small package. The seeds contain plant compounds called phytosterols and potent antioxidants which help combat many known diseases.

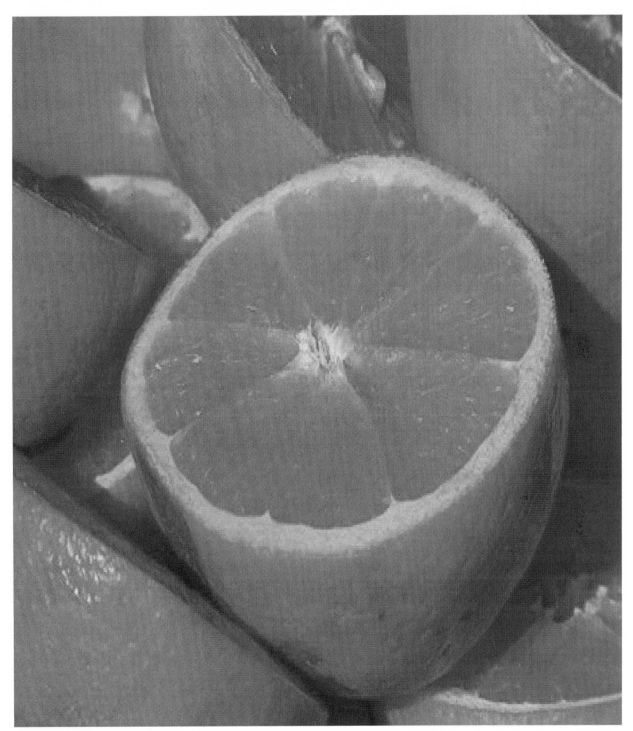

Orange

Oranges are natural source of several vitamins and minerals, notably vitamin C, thiamin, foliate and potassium. Vitamin C found in *Oranges* are a perfect source of vitamin C. One big *orange* can give more than 100% of the daily recommended needs.

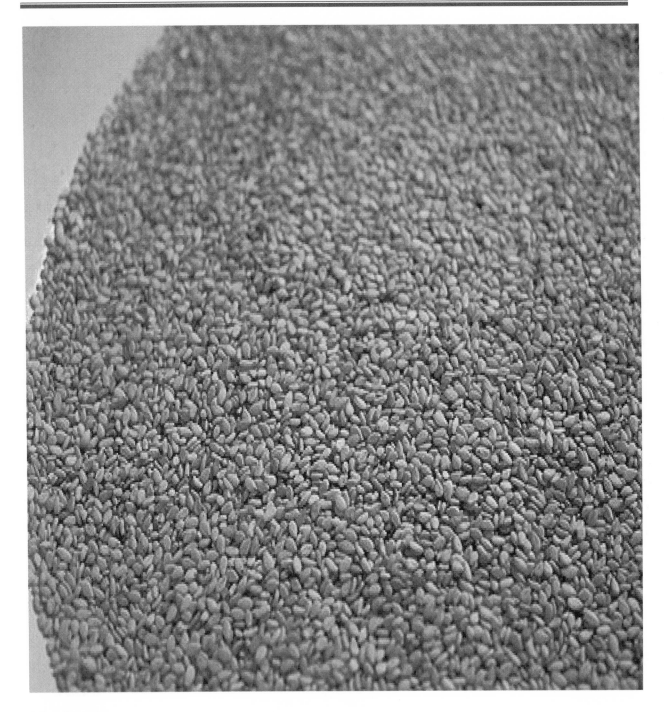

Mustard

Mustard is a micro seeds that have about 35 *calories*, 2.6 grams of protein, 2.2 grams of fat and 2.6 grams of carbohydrate in each portion of two teaspoons. The seeds also contain *dietary* fiber when consumed whole, having 1 gram or 4 percent of the recommended daily *needs*.

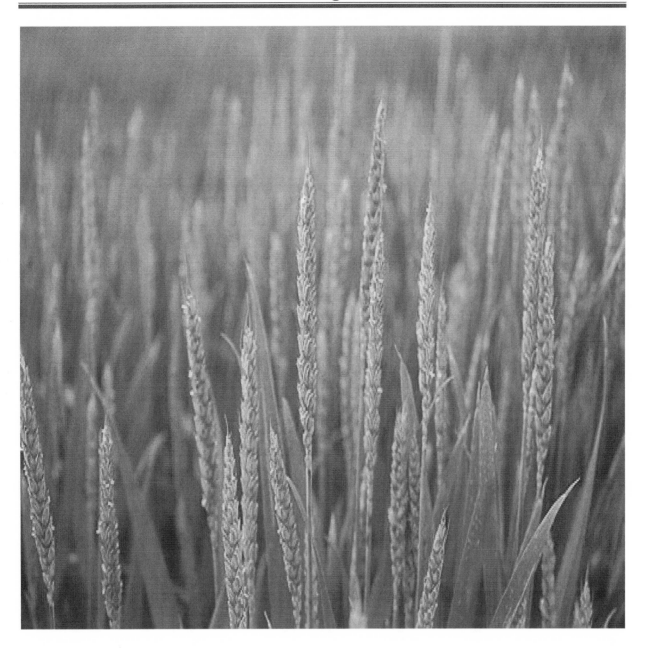

Licorice

Licorice lots of beneficial nutrients and flavonoids. It is an excellent source of thiamine, riboflavin, niacin, pantothenic acid and vitamin E, phosphorous, calcium, iron, magnesium, potassium, selenium, silicon and zinc.

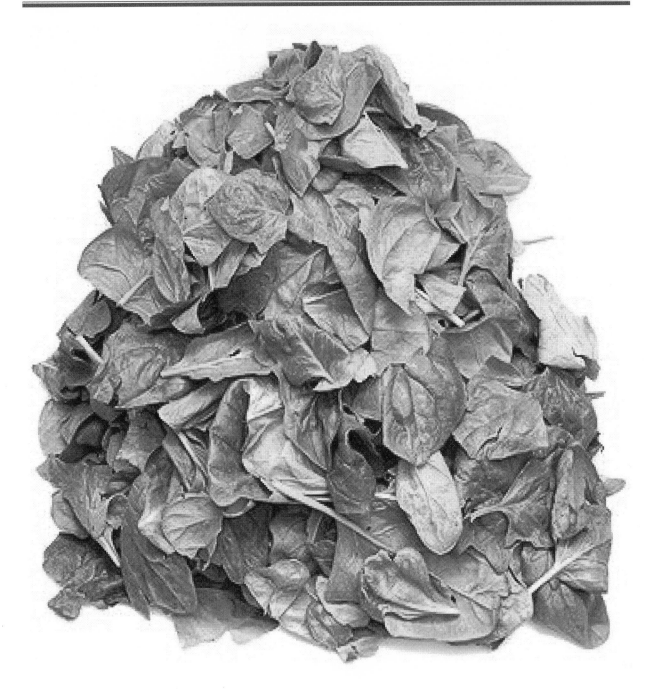

Spinach

Spinach is a good source of *vitamin K*, vitamin A, manganese, magnesium, iron, copper, vitamin B2, vitamin B6, vitamin E, calcium, potassium and vitamin C. It is rich in dietary fiber, phosphorus, vitamin B1, zinc, protein and chorine.

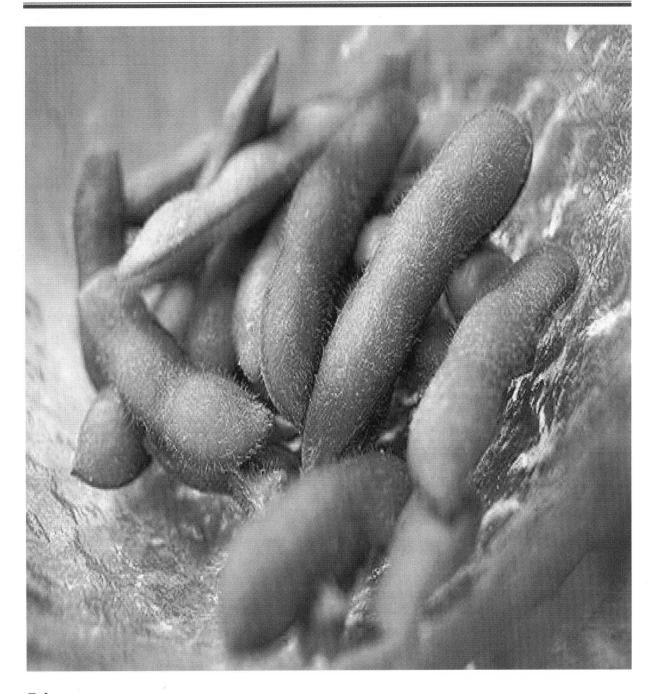

Edamame

Edamame are dense of nutrition. One cup a daily is enough to meet daily's needs. It is low in Sodium and a good source of *Dietary* Fiber, Protein, Thiamin, Iron, Magnesium, Phosphorus, Copper, Vitamin K, Foliate and Manganese.

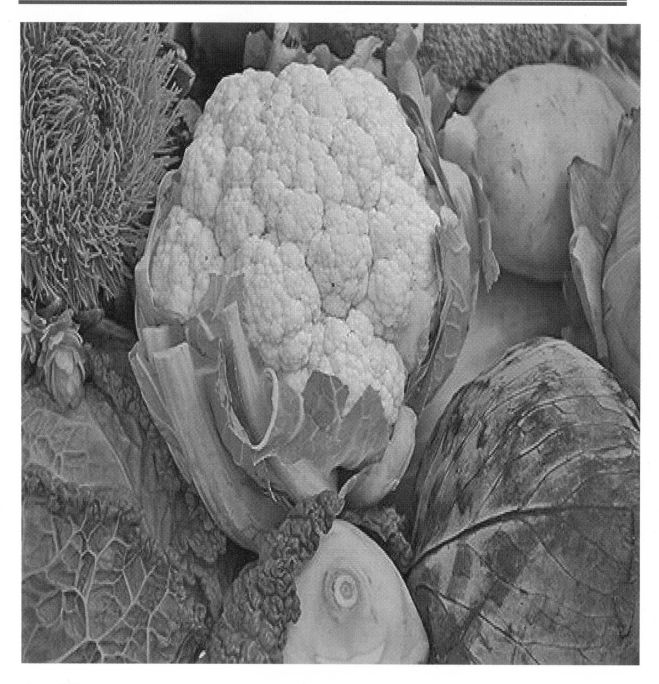

Cauliflower

Cauliflower is a good source of Protein, Niacin, Thiamin, Riboflavin, Magnesium and Phosphorus, and also contains an excellent *Dietary* Fiber, Vitamin C, Vitamin K, Vitamin B6, Potassium and Manganese. Cauliflower also has a special composition called glucosinolates which activate detoxification enzymes.

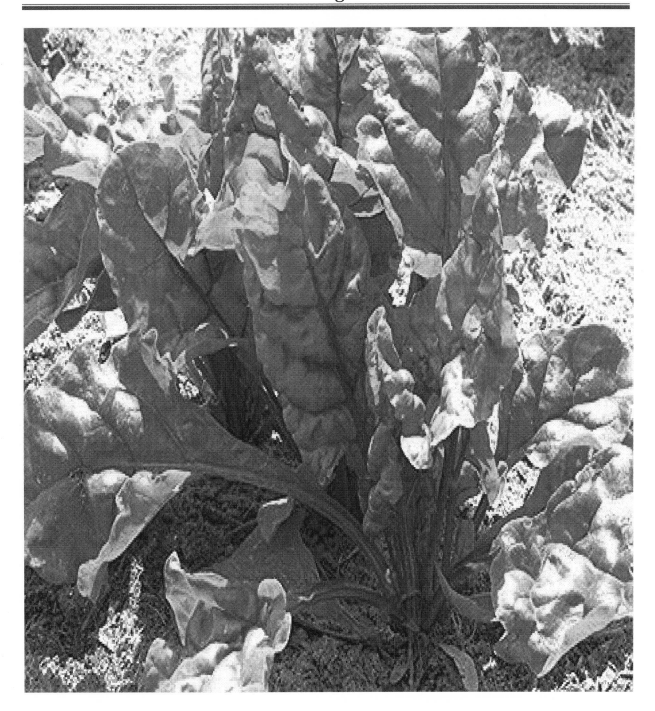

Swiss chard

Swiss chard is rich in vitamin K, vitamin A, vitamin C, magnesium, copper, manganese, potassium, vitamin E and iron, *dietary* fiber, vitamin B2, calcium, vitamin B6, phosphorus and protein. It's a leafy green vegetable and power bank of many phytonutrients that have health promotional and disease prevention properties.

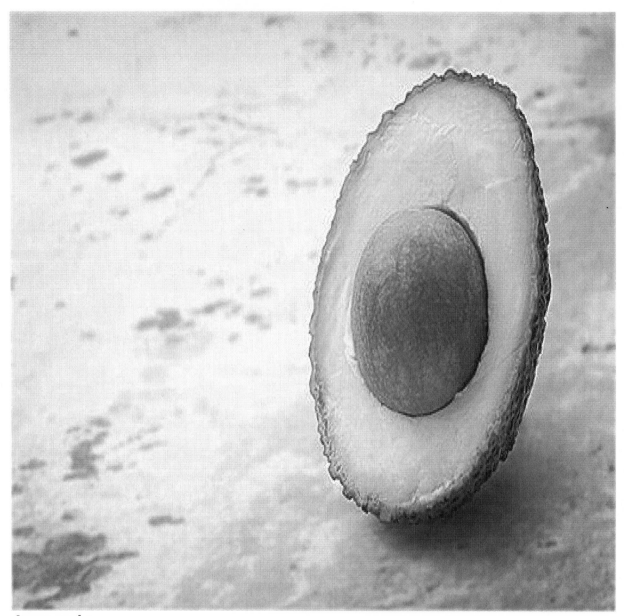

Avocado

Avocado is a succulent and highly *nutritious* fruit. It contain large amount of healthy fats, fiber, potassium and antioxidants with numerous health *benefits*.

Avocados are rich in *dietary* fiber, vitamin K, copper, foliate, vitamin B6, potassium, vitamin E, and vitamin C. Avocados fat *content* is between 71 to 88% of their total *calories*—which is 20 times the average for many other fruits.

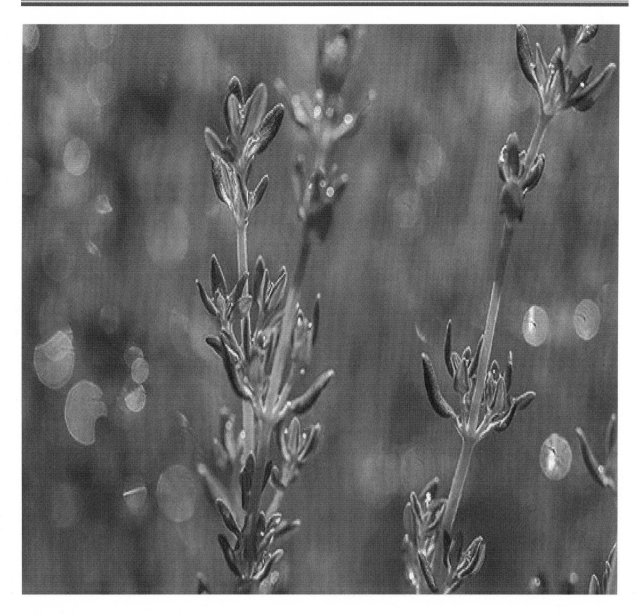

Thyme

Thyme is dense in minerals and vitamins that are excellent for a good health. Thyme leaves are rich in potassium, iron, calcium, manganese, magnesium, and selenium. Potassium presence in thyme helps to control heart rate and blood pressure. The manganese presence acts as an antioxidant enzyme which is good in fighting cancer. Thyme contains many more active ingredients that help in disease prevention.

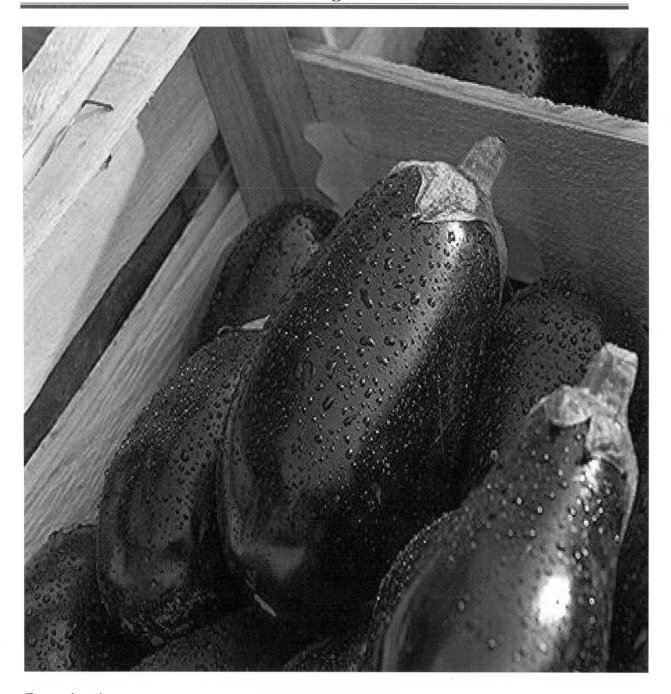

Eggplant

Eggplant is an excellent source of *dietary* fiber, vitamin B1 and copper, manganese, vitamin B6, niacin, potassium, foliate and vitamin K. *Eggplant* also has phytonutrients such as nasunin and chlorogenic acid. *Eggplant has the antioxidants properties that* support heart health, fight cancer and maintain weight and cholesterol level.

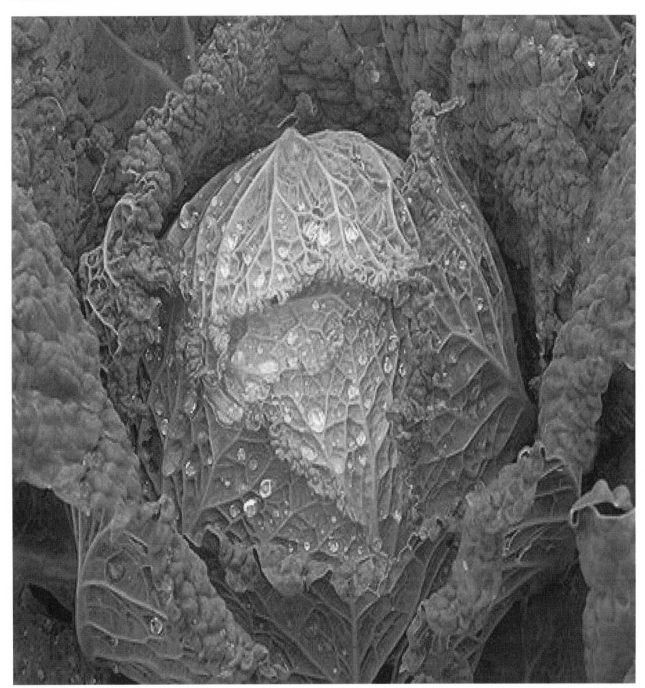

Cabbage

Cabbage is low in Sodium, Saturated Fat and Cholesterol. It is a rich source of Thiamin, Magnesium and Phosphorus, *Dietary* Fiber, Vitamin C, Vitamin K, Vitamin B6, Foliate, Calcium, Potassium and Manganese. It is a good food in fighting cancer, lower blood sugar, control blood pressure and some other ailments.

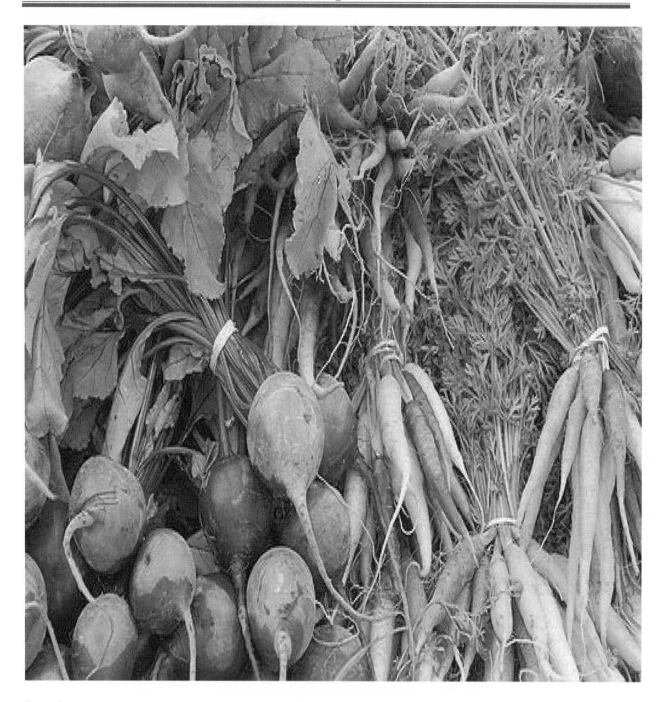

Beets

Beetroot s is a highly *nutritional plant* and is rich in calcium, iron and vitamins A and C. Beetroots are a perfect source of folic

Research has shown that beetroot has the ability to ward off cancer and also beet extract has been successfully used in treating human pancreatic, breast, and prostate cancers.

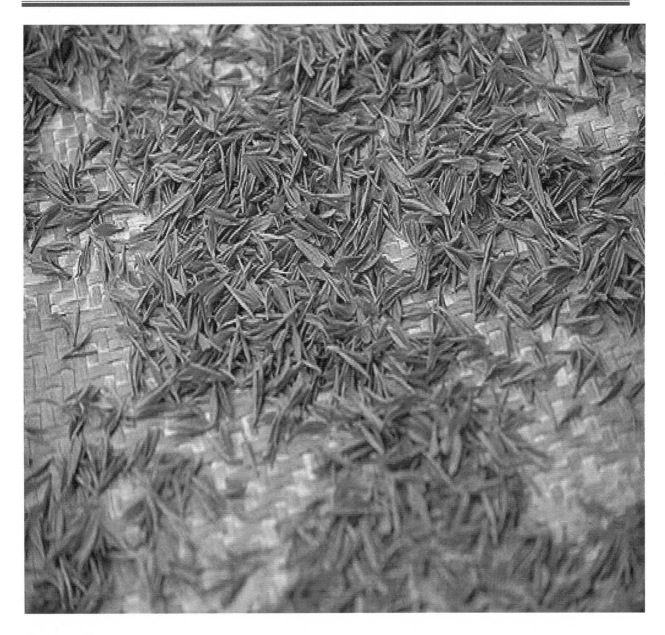

Green Tea

Green tea is loaded with antioxidants and nutrients that have powerful body effects. It is loaded with flavonoids and catechins, which function as strong antioxidants .The substance in green tea can lower the formation of free radicals in the body thereby protecting the cells and molecules from damage. These free radicals are known to be a big player in aging and all sorts of diseases. This includes improved brain function, fat loss, a lower risk of cancer and so many others.

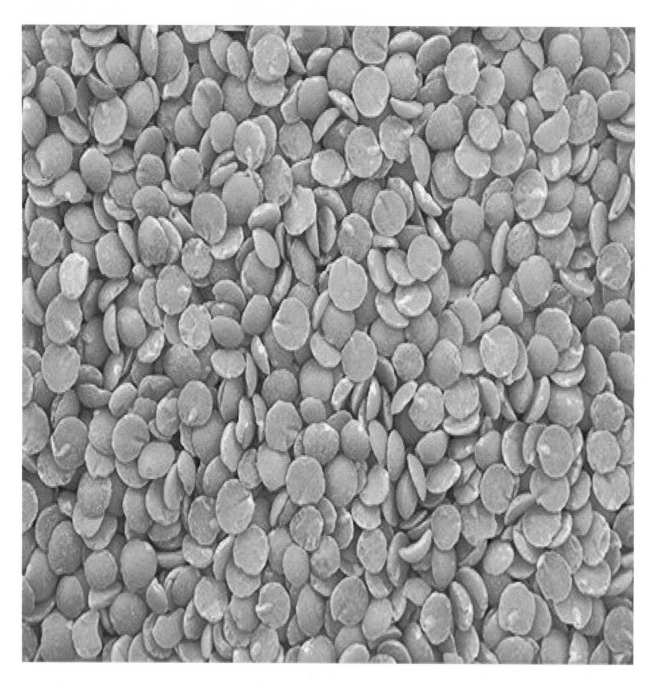

Lentils

Lentils are an excellent source of *dietary* fiber, copper, phosphorus and manganese, molybdenum and foliate. Furthermore, they are a perfect source of zinc, iron, protein, vitamin B1, potassium and vitamin B6.

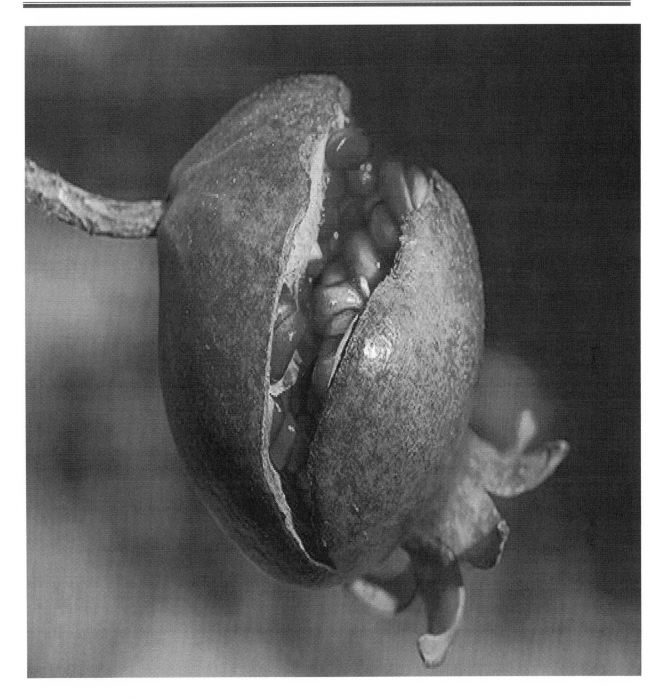

Pomegranates

Pomegranates are rich in soluble and insoluble *dietary* fibers with moderate calories and no cholesterol presence. Study has shown that pomegranate extract was found to prevent the growth of human breast cancer cells by inducing cell death.

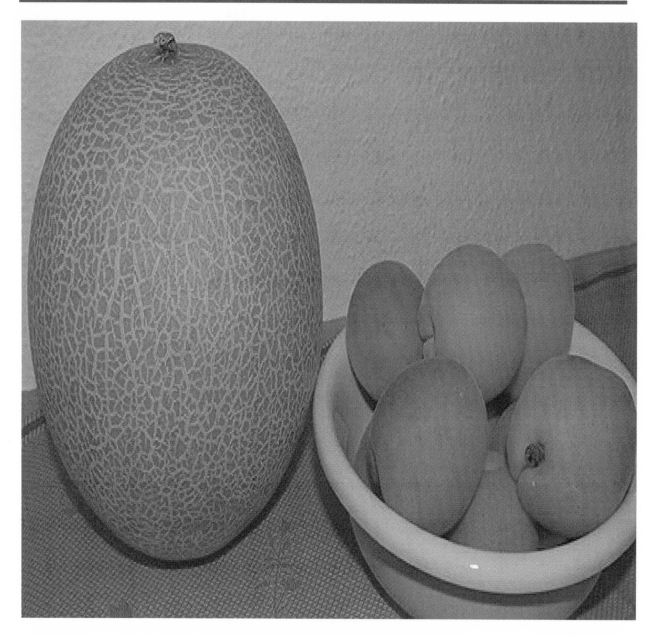

Apricot

Apricot is one of the world cleanness and healthiest food with lots of benefits. It is a god source of vitamin A, vitamin C, copper, *dietary* fiber and potassium.

100 grams of fresh apricots contain; 12% of vitamin C, 12% of vitamin A, 6% of potassium needed by the body – all this under less than 50 *calories*

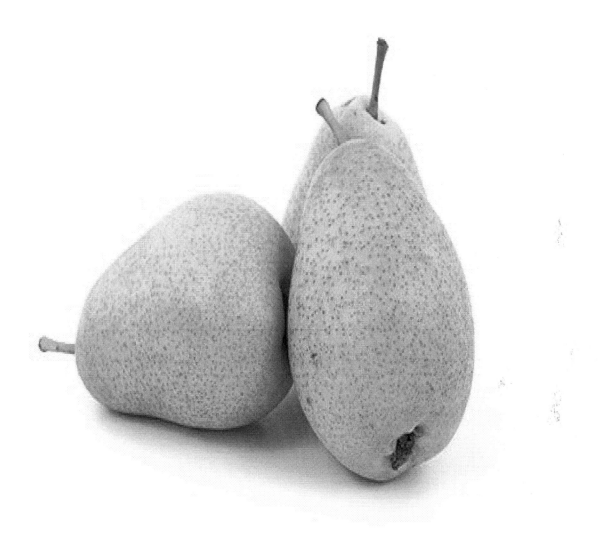

Pears

Pears are fruits that have low Saturated Fat, Cholesterol and Sodium. It is a good source of Vitamin C, and *Dietary* Fiber.50% of the pears fiber is found on the skin. It helps in digestion, lower blood fat and cholesterol levels, and help moderate blood sugar as well as in the treatment of cancer.

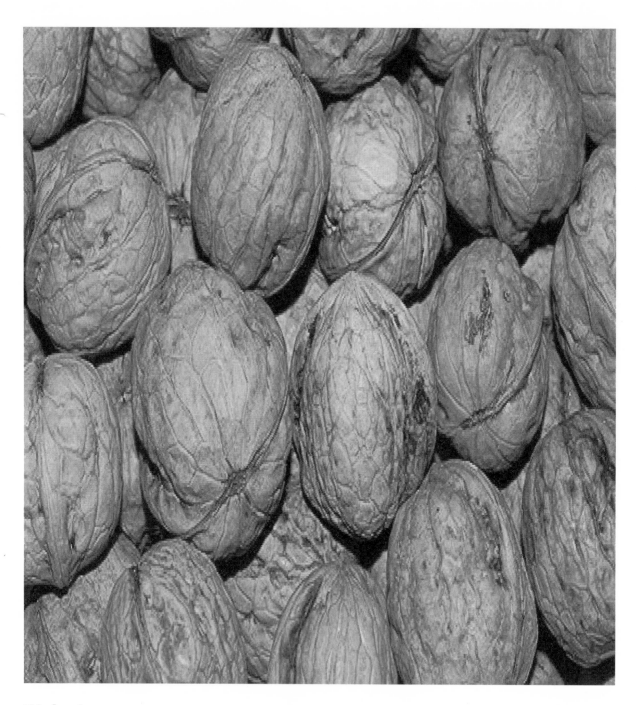

Walnuts

Walnuts are good source of anti-inflammatory omega-3 essential fatty acids, manganese, copper, molybdenum and the B vitamin biotin. *It is* excellently rich in antioxidants that help to fight so many diseases.

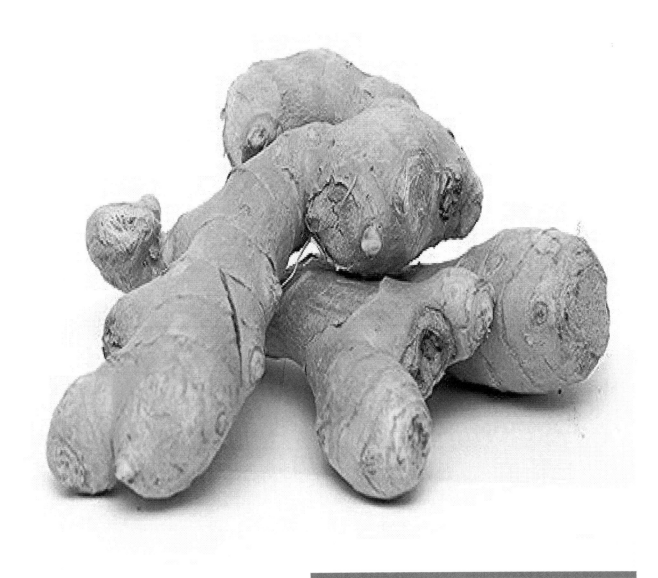

Ginger

Ginger is low in Saturated Fat, Cholesterol and Sodium and a good source of Vitamin C, Magnesium, Potassium, and Copper. The main active compound in ginger is called gingerol which gives provides much of the medicinal value.

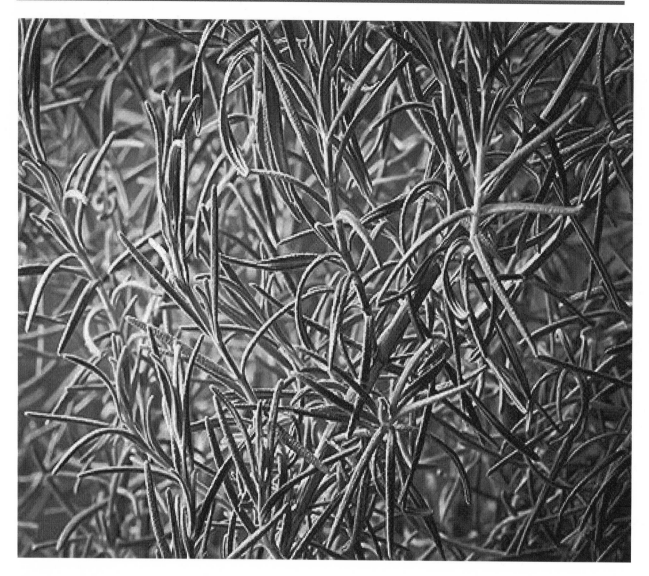

Rosemary

Rosemary contain a lots of *health benefits*. It is a good source of iron, calcium, and dietary fiber with presence of powerful antioxidants which helps to combat various ailments.

The dried *rosemary* provides;

93 *calories*,

12 grams of fiber and

45% of the daily *value* in iron,

35% of the calcium,

29% of the vitamin C and

18% of the vitamin **A** required

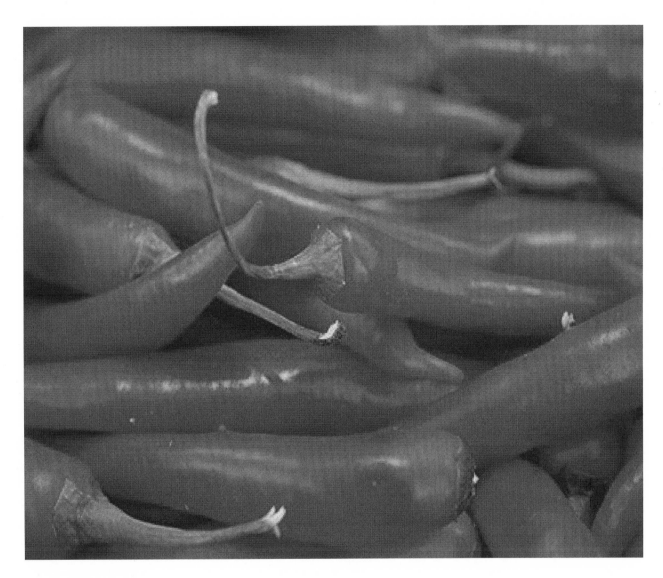

Chili Peppers

Chili peppers, despite their fiery hotness, are one of the very popular spices known for their *medicinal* and health benefiting *properties*.

This food is low in Sodium, and very low in Saturated Fat and Cholesterol. It is also a good source of *Dietary* Fiber, Thiamin, Riboflavin, Niacin, Folate, Iron, Magnesium, Phosphorus and Copper, and a very good source of Vitamin A, Vitamin C, Vitamin K, Vitamin B6, Potassium and Manganese.

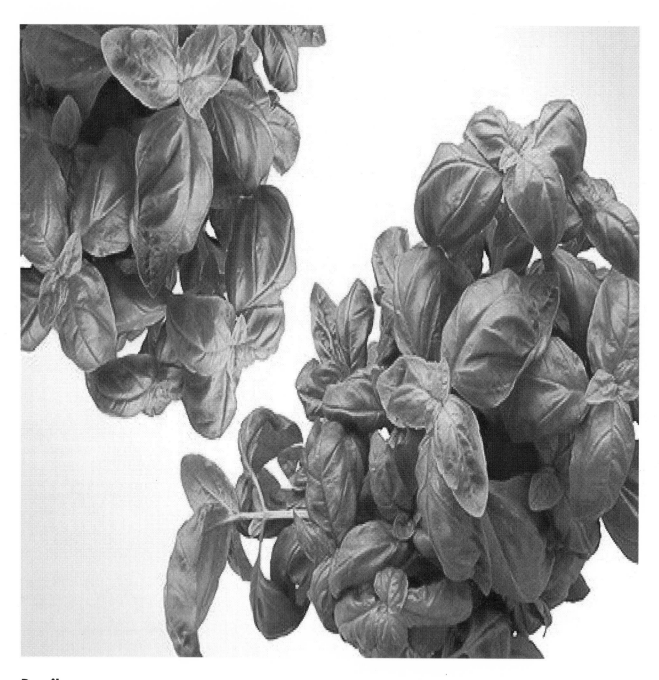

Basil

Basil is rich in Protein, Vitamin E, Riboflavin and Niacin, and are an excellent source of *Dietary* Fiber, Vitamin A, Vitamin C, Vitamin K, Vitamin B6, Foliate, Calcium, Iron, Magnesium, Phosphorus, Potassium, Zinc, Copper and Manganese. It is a strong herb that is highly medicinal and possesses ability to fight many ailments.

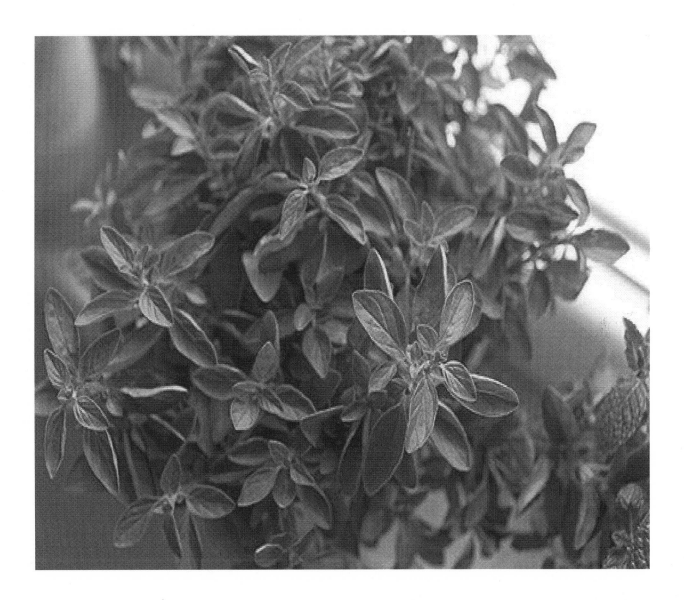

Oregano

Oregano is an important medicinal herb loaded with antioxidants. It is cholesterol free and are rich source of *dietary* fiber, that helps to regulate blood cholesterol levels. *Oregano* has many health benefiting oils loke; carvacrol, thymol and limonene. *Oregano*'s leaves are a good source of vitamin K, manganese, iron, *dietary* fiber and calcium.

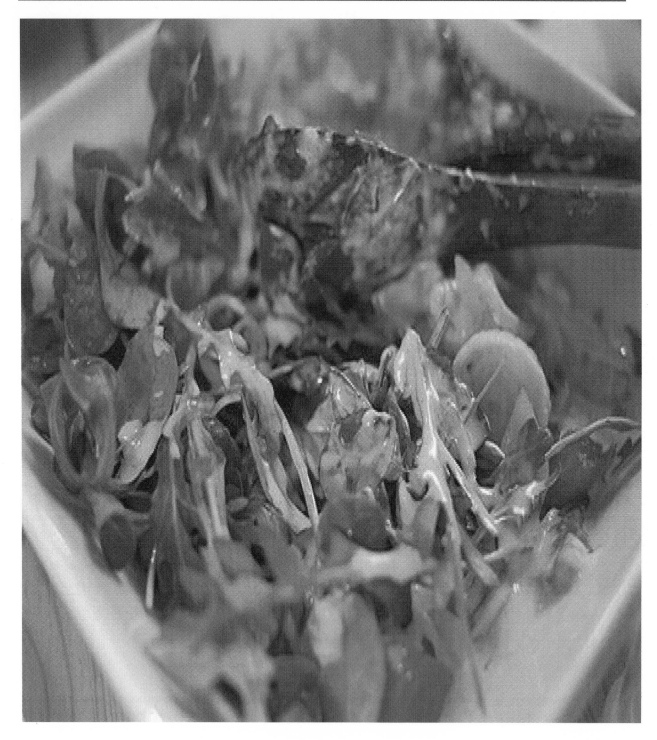

Arugula salads

Arugula is a fancy lettuce like veggie low in calorie.Its leaves are rich source of powerful phytochemicals which have been discovered to protect against prostate,breast,cervical,colon and ovarian cancers.

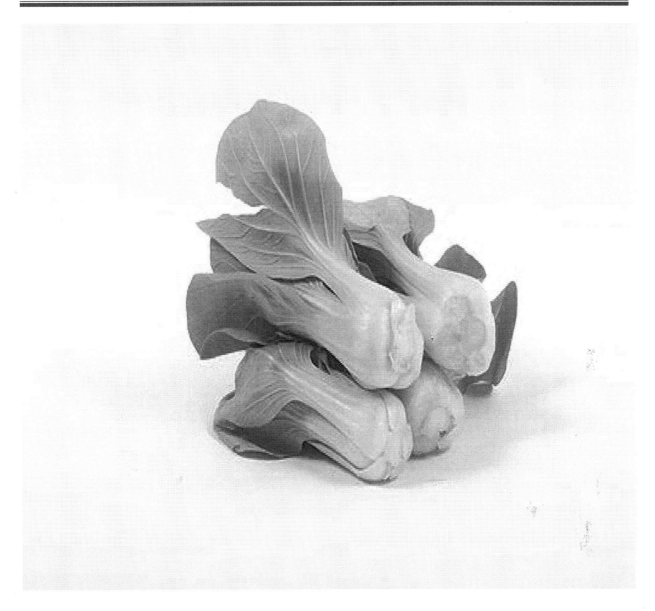

Bok choy

Bok choy is a veggie with a perfect source of vitamin K, vitamin C, vitamin A, potassium, *foliate*, vitamin B6, *calcium* and manganese. It many health benefits include; eliminating body fat, reduce blood sugar, control weight, fight cancer and many more.

A sizable litre of boy choy extract has about 9 calories, 1.5 gram of carbohydrates, 1 gram of protein, 0.7 grams of *dietary fiber*, and 0.1 grams of unsaturated fat and no cholesterol.

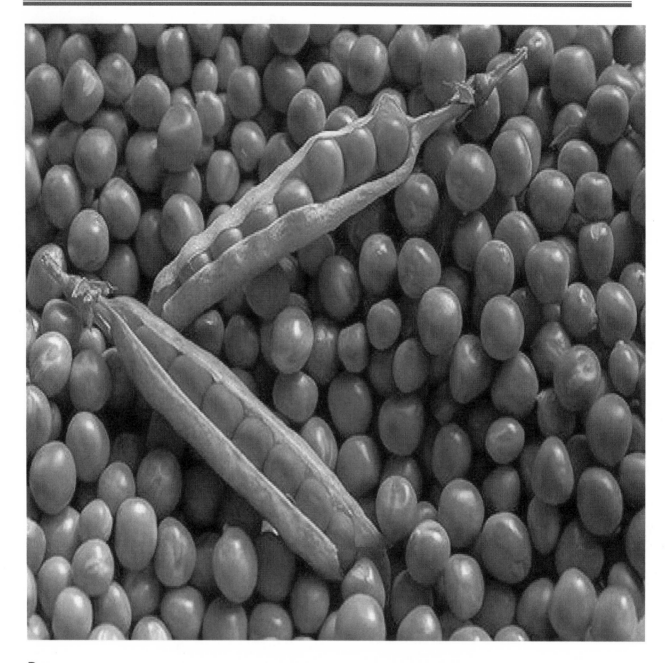

Peas

Peas are a food low in Saturated Fat, Cholesterol and Sodium. It is rich in *Protein*, Vitamin A, Riboflavin, Niacin, Vitamin B6, *Foliate*, Magnesium, Phosphorus and Copper, and an excellent source of *Dietary Fiber*, Vitamin C, Vitamin K, Thiamin and Manganese. It is useful in controlling diabetes, cancer and many other diseases.

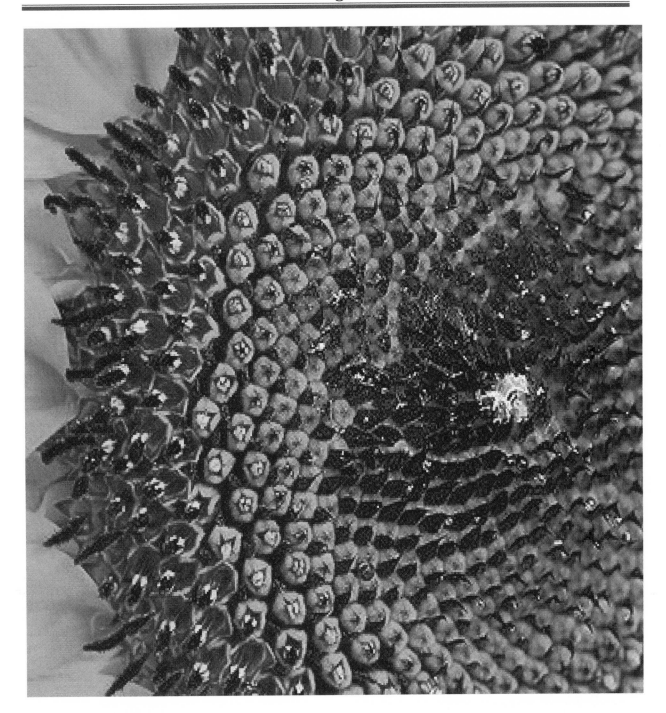

Sunflower seeds

Sunflower seeds are rich in vitamin E and an excellent source of copper and vitamin B1, manganese, selenium, phosphorus, magnesium, vitamin B6, foliate and niacin. The oil in the sunflower is powerful antioxidants that fight to curbs many diseases.

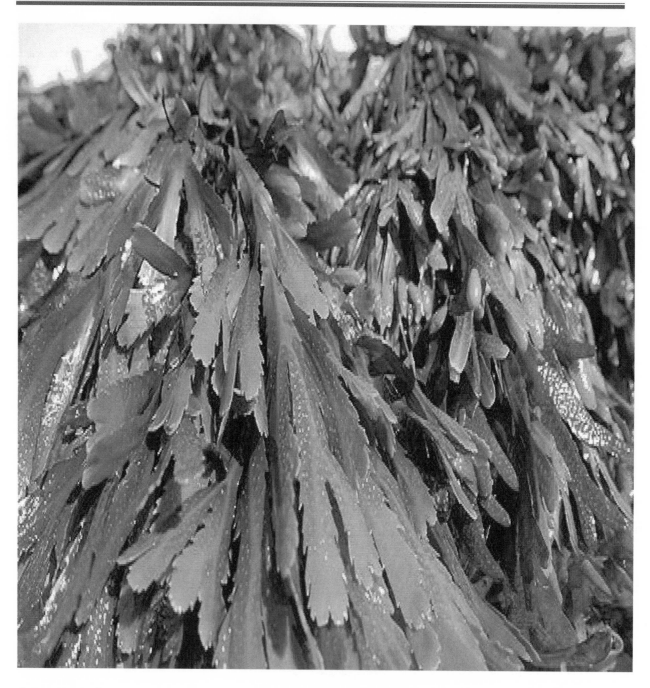

Seaweed

Seaweed is blessed with low Saturated Fat, and very low Cholesterol. It is rich in Vitamin A, Vitamin C, Vitamin E, Vitamin K, Niacin, Phosphorus, Riboflavin, Foliate, Calcium, Iron, Magnesium, Copper and Manganese. It is highly medicinal with strong antioxidants.

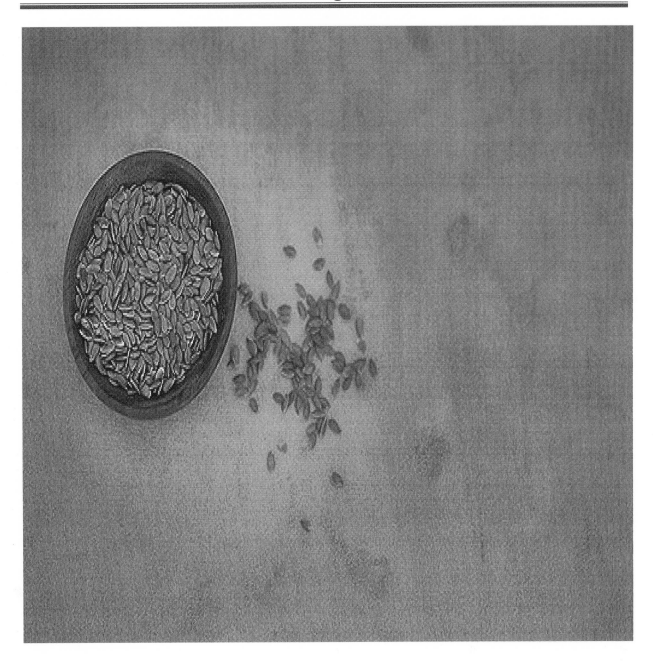

Flax seeds

Flaxseeds are very rich in omega-3 essential fatty acids and a perfect source of dietary fiber, vitamin B1, copper, minerals magnesium, phosphorus and selenium. Flax seed has numerous benefits which includes; improve digestion, lower cholesterol level, balance hormones, fight cancer and promote weight loss and many more.

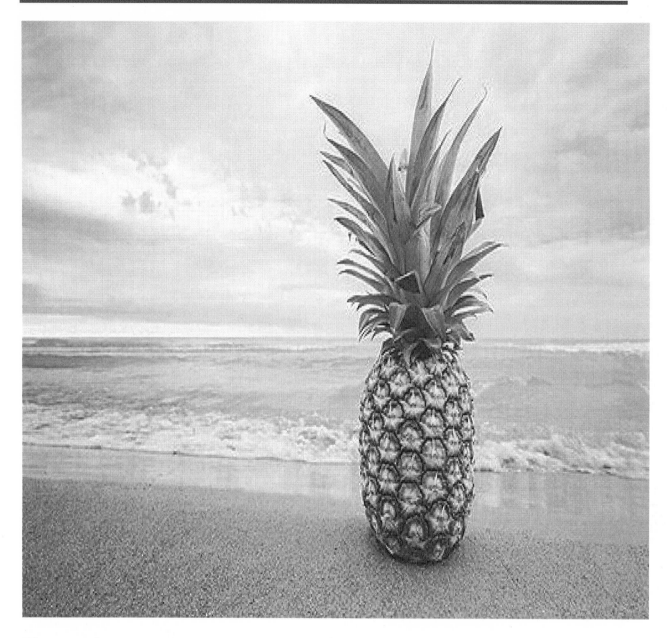

Pineapple

Pineapples are tropical fruits and are a good source of many nutrients, such as *vitamin C*, manganese, copper and foliate. Pineapples also contain plant compound called bromelain which has many positive effect on human lives.

Carbs: 13.1 g   **Protein**: 0.5 g

Calories: 50   **Sugar**: 9.9 g

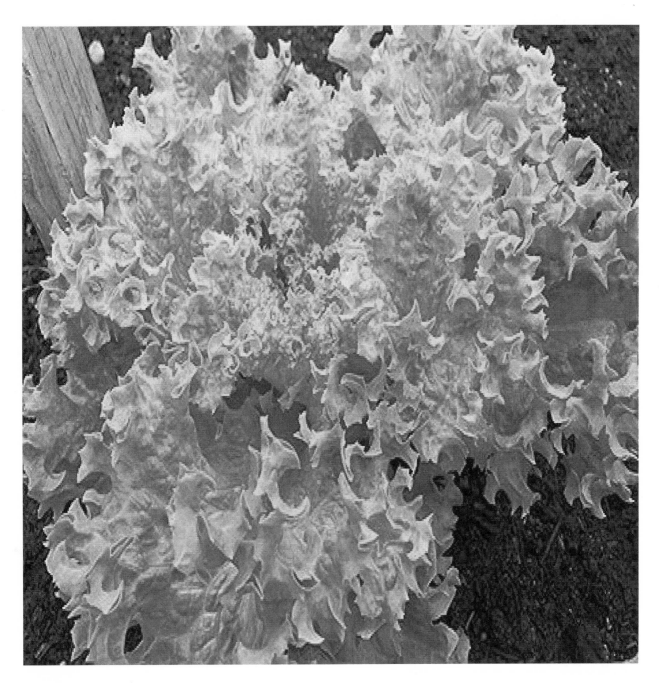

Endive

Endive is green leafy vegetable also known as escarole. It is rich in Vitamin E, Magnesium and Phosphorus, *dietary* Fiber, Vitamin A, Vitamin C, Vitamin K, Thiamin, Riboflavin, Foliate, Calcium, Iron, Potassium, Zinc, Copper and Manganese.

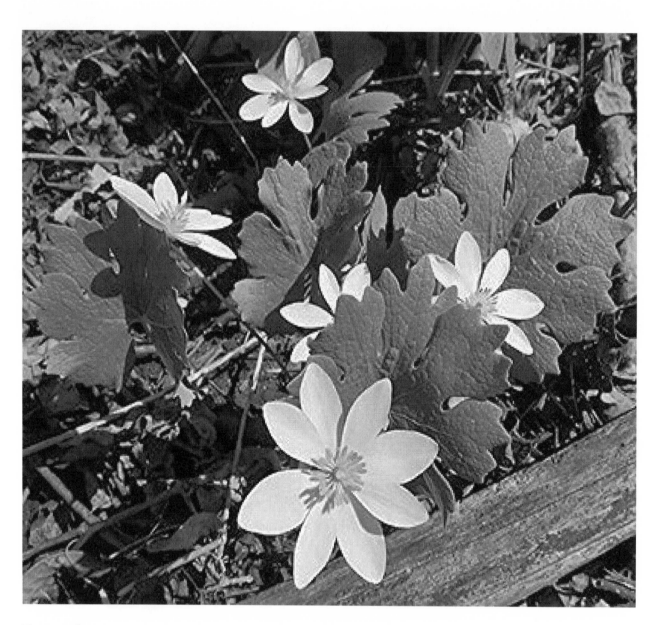

Tumeric

Turmeric is a good source of iron and manganese. It is also rich in vitamin B6, *dietary* fiber, copper, and potassium. Some of the health benefits of turmeric include its ability to heal wound, alleviate pain, slow the aging process, prevent cancer and many more.

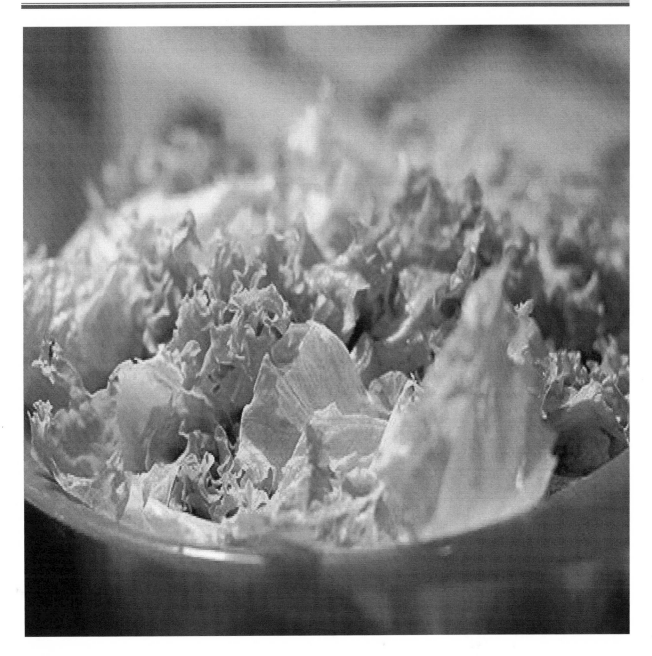

Lettuce

Lettuce contains a powerful antioxidants and nutrients that helps in promoting good health and act as a disease prevention *properties*

Lettuce has low Saturated Fat and Cholesterol. It is rich in Protein, Calcium, Magnesium and Phosphorus, *Dietary* Fiber, Vitamin A, Vitamin C, Vitamin K, Thiamin, Riboflavin, Vitamin B6, Foliate, Iron, Potassium and Manganese.

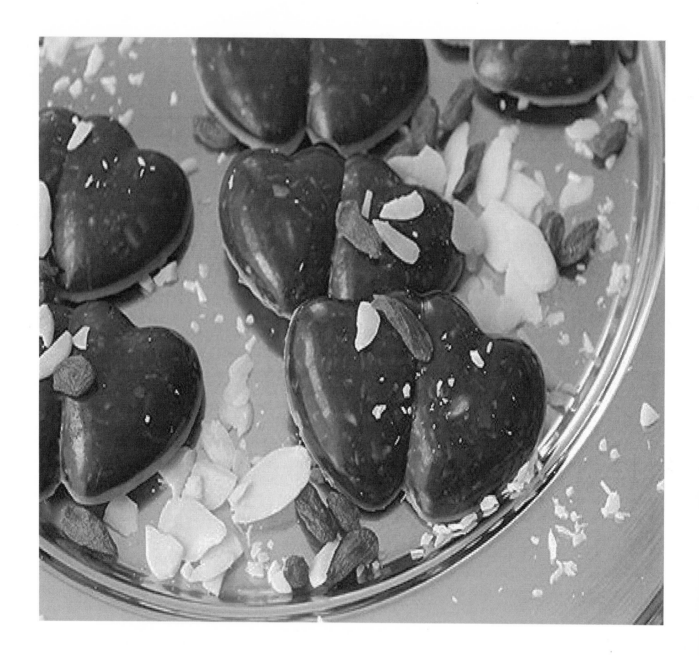

GOJI

Goji berries are one of world healthiest dried fruits because of their high antioxidant *content*, which aid a longer lifespan. It is low in Sodium, Saturated Fat and Cholesterol and also rich in Protein, Thiamin and Calcium, *Dietary* Fiber, Vitamin A, Vitamin C, Riboflavin, Iron, Potassium, Zinc, Copper and Selenium.

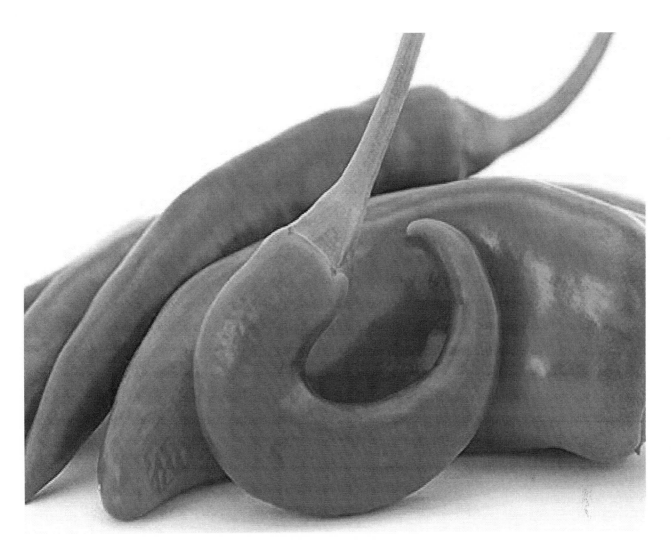

Jalapenos

Jalapenos are low in Saturated Fat, Cholesterol and Sodium. It is rich in Riboflavin, Niacin, Iron, Magnesium, Phosphorus, *Dietary* Fiber, Vitamin A, Vitamin C, Vitamin K, Thiamin, Vitamin B6, Foliate, Potassium, Copper and Manganese

Jalapeno pepper is good in treating stomach ulcer, weight loss, clear sinuses, treating migraine, cancer and many more.

Other book from the Author

Herbal Remedies: Foods As Medicine Approach. A
Nature Cure for Illnesses

Get it here: getbook.at/Foodasmedicine

Made in the USA
Middletown, DE
18 May 2019